"This is a valuable book that comes at a critical time, when digital health has accelerated across the globe fanned by the fire of the pandemic. It provides an informed account of the factors to consider and practical steps to make the most of the opportunity."
– **Tara Donelly,** *Founder, Digital Care, Ex-Chief Digital Officer, NHS Digital*

"Digital healthcare is not merely a subset of traditional healthcare; it represents a reconfiguration of the entire healthcare system. Therefore, any effort to digitally transform organisations and effectively prepare them for the future must adopt an ecosystem approach. This book offers a practical framework for implementing this approach, highlighting the necessity for collective action as no single organisation can undertake this transformation alone."
– **Jorge Armanet,** *Entrepeneur, Operator Investor and Advisor*
Founder and Former CEO of HealthUnlocked
Cambridge Digital Innovation Fellow

"This book gives excellent insight into the benefits, risks and their mitigation of the use of digital technologies in healthcare. It then covers proposals on how we should regulate and respond to these new technologies to avoid the risks this new paradigm brings. I would recommend this book to anyone working in digital healthcare."
– **Stephen Critchlow,** *Founder, CEO and Chair of*
Wellbeing Team at Evergreen Life, Chair of the
NIHR AI in Healthcare Board

"This book illustrates the key changes in the industry when COVID-19 accelerated digital healthcare. When I first presented patient portals in the UK it was something the NHS could not see would be used or adopted. Data silos cause so much complexity and create gaps in patient records. As these challenges are addressed we start to see the value being created and this is a process explored in this book. The book offers a comprehensive understanding of the complexity of digital transformation in healthcare."
– **Chris Rushworth,** *Head of Product, Doctor Care Anywhere*

"This is an important book. We are facing a global health crisis and the current 'egosystem' approach is never going to scale and offer the right economics to address the global need. This book illustrates how digital technologies can create and transform health ecosystems in way that was never possible and how these digital arenas change the economics of the market allowing greater participation and delivering additional value to those participants. The framework it offers provides a pragmatic guide to the journey to this ecosystem model, allowing the reader to embark on the journey without the associated risks such undertakings often attract. Highly recommended."
us Robbins, *Chief Digital Advisor – Head of Strategy*
and Growth – DX Services – Fujitsu UK

"This rich and engaging book about contemporary challenges in healthcare offers a unique perspective. Targeting practitioners and managers, it operationalises key insights from otherwise hard-to-get academic discussions by carefully selecting, presenting and illustrating these in accessible form – without trivialising them."

– **Eric Monteiro**, *Professor of Information Systems,*
Norwegian University of Science and Technology

"Professor Constantinides brilliantly navigates healthcare's digital transformation using powerful concepts and vivid examples. His framework illuminates how ecosystem strategy, technology, and human resources empower diverse actors to co-innovate and co-create value. Thoughtfully balancing the possibilities and risks of disruptive technologies like Generative AI and blockchain, he provides an indispensable roadmap for this evolving landscape. A must-read for anyone vested in the future of healthcare!"

– **Arun Rai**, *Regents' Professor and Howard S. Starks Distinguished Chair,*
Georgia State University

"*Digital Transformation in Healthcare: An Ecosystem Approach* by Professor Constantinides expertly traverses the healthcare landscape. Highlighting the importance of partnerships, digital platforms, and an ecosystem perspective, it offers strategic co-innovation insights for value creation. The book incisively illuminates the potentials of Generative AI, learning infrastructures, and blockchain technologies. An indispensable guide, the book offers profound insights into digital transformation for anyone in healthcare."

– **Elena Karahanna**, *Distinguished Research Professor and*
C. Herman & Mary Virginia Terry Distinguished Chair
in Business Administration, University of Georgia

"In *Digital Transformation in Healthcare: An Ecosystem Approach*, Panos Constantinides provides much-needed guidance for healthcare managers, indeed all managers. He takes a 'show, don't tell' approach by methodically showing the steps, with examples, that organizations must follow to digitally transform their operations and strategy. The ecosystem approach is necessary for the future success of healthcare organizations so that they can focus on their core competency of providing health services in an efficient and effective manner."

– **Rajiv Kohli**, *John N. Dalton Memorial Professor of Business,*
Raymond A. Mason School of Business, William & Mary University

"Corporations tend to focus on the efficiency gains from digital transformation but, often, fail to see the real transformative power that digital technologies provide: the ability to re-imagine the new possible to achieve what most actors from the established value chain would consider impossible. This timely and comprehensive book is all about the 'impossible-new possible' in healthcare through digital transformation, and the enabling role played by digital technologies and ecosystems.

Panos Constantinides presents a compelling framework for healthcare organizations to navigate the complex landscape of digital transformation. From telemedicine and blockchain to federated learning and generative AI technologies, this book provides a rich journey into how ecosystem approaches can activate collaborative partnerships and collective action to unlock innovation and drive transformative change in healthcare solutions. It is a 'must read' for healthcare organizations, policymakers, and empowered patients alike who want to shape the new possible."

— **Carmelo Cennamo,** *Professor, Copenhagen Business School*

"*Digital Transformation in Healthcare: An Ecosystem Approach* tackles some of the most complex challenges in a critical industry and carefully develops the what, why, and how. Using concrete examples, the book lays out the key value propositions and architecture, makes the case for the need to change, and develops actionable strategies to make it happen while managing the risks and governance challenges that are sure to arise. I highly recommend it as a key manual to create positive change in healthcare."

— **Geoffrey Parker,** *Charles E. Hutchinson '68A Professor of Engineering Innovation, Dartmouth College, co-author of* Platform Revolution

Digital Transformation in Healthcare

In an era of digital transformation within healthcare management, this important book outlines an ecosystem perspective to illustrate how a range of actors can use digital technologies to offer better value within the provision of healthcare services.

From mobile applications to point-of-care diagnostic devices, from AI-enabled applications for data analysis to cloud models for service delivery and blockchain infrastructures, it provides a roadmap for how healthcare organizations can leverage these digital technologies. The book is also illustrated with case studies from different areas, including software for medical diagnostics, blockchain infrastructures for use in pharmaceutical supply chains and clinical trials, and federated learning platforms for genomics.

Covering key issues such as patients' rights to data and written in the aftermath of the COVID-19 pandemic, the book will be essential reading for researchers, postgraduate students and professionals interested in how technology can support and enable healthcare service provision.

Panos Constantinides is Professor of Digital Innovation and Digital Learning Lead for Executive Education at Alliance Manchester Business School. He is also a Fellow of the Cambridge Digital Innovation Centre. His research focuses on the transformative potential of digital technology, including digital platforms, infrastructures and artificial intelligence. His research has been published in both academic journals and media outlets.

Digital Transformation in Healthcare

An Ecosystem Approach

Panos Constantinides

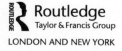

LONDON AND NEW YORK

Designed cover image: Costas Constantinides

First published 2024
by Routledge
4 Park Square, Milton Park, Abingdon, Oxon OX14 4RN

and by Routledge
605 Third Avenue, New York, NY 10158

Routledge is an imprint of the Taylor & Francis Group, an informa business

British Library Cataloguing-in-Publication Data
A catalogue record for this book is available from the British Library

Library of Congress Cataloguing-in-Publication Data
Names: Constantinides, Panos, author.
Title: Digital transformation in healthcare : an ecosystem approach /
Panos Constantinides.
Description: Abingdon, Oxon ; New York, NY : Routledge, 2024. |
Includes bibliographical references and index.
|Identifiers: LCCN 2023029331 | ISBN 9781032619576 (hbk) | ISBN 9781032171111 (pbk) | ISBN 9781032619569 (ebk)
Subjects: LCSH: Medical informatics. | Medical informatics--Technological innovations. | Medicine--Data processing. | Medical care.
Classification: LCC R858 .C6645 2024 | DDC 610.285--dc23/eng/20230925
LC record available at https://lccn.loc.gov/2023029331

ISBN: 978-1-032-61957-6 (hbk)
ISBN: 978-1-032-17111-1 (pbk)
ISBN: 978-1-032-61956-9 (ebk)

DOI: 10.4324/9781032619569

Typeset in Sabon
by MPS Limited, Dehradun

Contents

Preface

In recent years, the world has experienced significant disruption by such major shocks as the COVID-19 pandemic, but also the coming of age of generative AI, both of which have accelerated digital transformation. The COVID-19 pandemic has highlighted the urgent need for digital solutions that can improve patient outcomes, increase operational efficiency and ensure access to healthcare services. The pandemic has forced healthcare organizations to rapidly adopt digital solutions, such as telemedicine and remote monitoring, to ensure continuity of care and reduce the risk of infection. As a result, the adoption of digital health solutions has accelerated significantly, and many of these changes are likely to become permanent. In addition, the rapid pace of technological change through digital technologies such as artificial intelligence, cloud computing and the Internet of Medical Things but also biotechnologies such as mRNA and whole genome sequencing has enabled the development of new digital health solutions, most notably in personalized or precision medicine, which were not possible a decade ago. Patients are becoming more active and empowered in managing their own health and wellness through personal smart devices and they are putting significant pressure on healthcare service providers to become more efficient and effective.

The need for a book on digital transformation in healthcare is more urgent now than ever before. Disruptive forces are transforming the healthcare sector in fundamental ways that require executives in healthcare organizations to be more proactive and strategic in their approach to digital transformation.

Much of this digital transformation is felt in developed economies, including the UK, the European Union, the USA and China, among others, where most research and development in new technological solutions is taking place. However, developing economies can also benefit from digital transformation in healthcare, even if most of the research and development in new technological solutions is taking place elsewhere. Digital technologies, such as telemedicine, can help overcome geographic barriers and improve access to healthcare services in developing economies. Patients in rural areas, for example, may have limited access to healthcare facilities and specialists, but can benefit from telemedicine consultations with doctors in urban areas. Digital technologies can help improve the quality of care in developing economies by enabling healthcare professionals to access up-to-date medical information, and collaborate with specialists and monitor patients remotely through virtual wards. This can help reduce medical errors and improve patient outcomes. Digital technologies can also help reduce healthcare costs in developing economies by improving efficiency and reducing the need for costly infrastructures. For example, remote patient monitoring can reduce the need for hospitalization and expensive medical equipment. Digital transformation in healthcare can also contribute to economic development in developing economies by creating new jobs and opportunities in the healthcare sector. It can also help attract foreign investment and improve the competitiveness of local businesses.

However, there are also challenges to implementing digital transformation in healthcare. These include limited resources, infrastructure and skills, as well as regulatory and cultural barriers. Indeed, these challenges are faced by healthcare organizations in both developing and developed economies. For example, a recent study in the English NHS found evidence of an "impending crisis, with capital restrictions limiting investment in buildings, infrastructure and equipment", all of which force the implementation of "rationing" practices, service dilution, delay and selection that impact the quality and safety of care. Many of these inefficiencies are due to the limitations of supply-driven forms of organizing healthcare services, including bureaucratic decision-making infused with political agendas. Such supply-driven forms of organizing drive up the costs of healthcare services including treatment options, diagnostics and hospital care. There is also a rising doctor and carer burnout across national health systems due to increased workloads, low numbers of staff and other resource constraints which contribute to medical errors and poor performance, feeding into a non-virtuous cycle of increased costs. These complex challenges are aggravated by the lack of interoperability between information systems and applications, as well as issues of data access. In addition, there are ethical and regulatory challenges to governing data generated through, and accessed by, new innovations in healthcare.

No single organization can navigate the complexity of the healthcare landscape on its own. No single organization has all the necessary resources and capabilities to innovate on its own. Rather, organizations need to develop collaborative partnerships with different actors to synergistically combine complementary resources and capabilities across healthcare ecosystems.

The key contribution of this book is a framework to help organizations leverage digital technologies across ecosystems in their transformation programs. Developing their own ecosystem or becoming a partner in other ecosystems is not simply about technology. It is about collaborating on complex problems and finding innovative solutions, establishing governance rules for managing risks and resolving collective action problems, and building joint value propositions that generate virtuous value creation opportunities for all ecosystem actors.

The book builds the rationale for an ecosystem approach to digital transformation, develops and applies the approach and discusses regulatory challenges over three parts and seven chapters. Part 1 sets the scene, with Chapter 1 reviewing the major forces disrupting healthcare services and defining key concepts, including disruption, digital transformation, digital maturity and ecosystems. This chapter discusses the emergence of multiple ecosystems, both small and large, and involving different ecosystem actors. Chapter 2 then provides a deep dive into the key challenges faced by healthcare organizations across the world, primarily because of the prevalence of supply-driven forms of organizing healthcare services. It provides examples of both incumbent organizations in the public and private sector, but also new startups and their efforts to manage challenges ranging from the rising costs of healthcare services, to interoperability challenges between diverse technologies, to ethical and regulatory challenges around data governance. Finally, Chapter 3 describes how organizations can lead change toward achieving higher value for patients. Value is discussed in relation to the healthcare delivery cycle, exploring how different ecosystem actors get involved in this cycle's distinct processes, going beyond healthcare service providers, to also examine the role of medical device manufacturers, diagnostic centers, biotech and pharmaceutical companies and digital service integrators, among others. Following this discussion, the focus shifts to how each of these ecosystem actors can develop unique value propositions by leveraging digital technologies. Chapter 3 outlines different levels of digital maturity, offering a blueprint by which healthcare organizations can identify where they stand and how they can begin to digitally transform themselves.

Part 2 is the core of the book providing a detailed discussion of the ecosystem approach to digital transformation. First, Chapter 4 lays out a framework of how organizations can digitally transform their services across an ecosystem, including how to define their digital transformation problem, clarify their incentives and activities, but also how to develop an innovation and adoption plan in collaboration with their partners, while governing associated risks. The chapter draws heavily on the example of the Siemens Healthineers' "teamplay digital health platform", which enables diverse organizations, from hospitals to diagnostic centres, to benefit from a modular, vendor-agnostic infrastructure and digital applications provided by third-party complementors on demand. The chapter discusses both the opportunities and collective action problems that may emerge in such ecosystems and also provides ways of effectively managing those while ensuring sustainability and growth. Chapter 5 discusses ways on how healthcare organizations can form ecosystems on blockchain infrastructures. This chapter describes how blockchain infrastructures work, how transactions take place and how they enable distributed data governance. It then provides a discussion of use cases of blockchain infrastructures in healthcare provided by PharmaLedger, focusing on recruiting patients and achieving informed consent in clinical trials, and achieving trusted transactions through electronic product information in pharmaceutical supply chains. The chapter concludes by discussing the co-innovation and co-adoption challenges of the use of blockchain infrastructures in healthcare. Chapter 6 discusses ways by which healthcare organizations can form ecosystems on federated learning infrastructures. The chapter describes how cloud computing works, before exploring data virtualization and federated learning infrastructures. It then discusses two use cases of federated learning in healthcare ecosystems, one in medical imaging used during the COVID-19 pandemic and one in genomics research hosted on the Lifebit platform. The chapter concludes by discussing the co-innovation and co-adoption challenges of the use of data virtualization in healthcare.

Part 3 concludes the book by discussing the recent coming of age of generative AI technologies, including OpenAI's Chat GPT-4, Microsoft's Bing AI and 365 Copilot, but also Meta's LLaMA and Google's Bard. Chapter 7 provides an analysis of this very turbulent landscape and discusses ways by which organizations can navigate digital transformation by using generative AI technologies. The chapter provides a discussion of both the possibilities and challenges of generative AI in healthcare, before diving deep into the race to tech arms between big tech companies, open-source developers and healthcare organizations. The chapter concludes by examining recent regulation on AI technologies and makes a set of proposals for technology policy to govern generative AI in healthcare.

I hope that the book provides a strategic blueprint for startups and incumbent organizations in healthcare to help them transform their operations and improve patient outcomes. Regulators and policy-makers but also empowered patients will also find the book useful in navigating the complexity of the healthcare landscape.

Panos Constantinides

Acknowledgments

This book is a lifelong product of thinking, conferring and writing on the topic of digital health. My interest in digital health is biased since I was born in a family of doctors. I remember myself as young as six years old, sitting at the kitchen table and listening to my dad, a neurosurgeon, and my mom, an anaesthesiologist, go over the details of operating on a patient with spondylolisthesis. Identifying symptoms and understanding how to deal with a disease were common conversation topics at the kitchen table, with myself and my siblings asking (mostly silly) questions, at least early on! Over time, my dad took on operational roles at the hospital where he worked, including becoming the hospital's President and later the Director for Clinical Governance. These roles helped to expand our conversations into organizational issues, including the use of new technologies across the healthcare delivery cycle. During this time, my brother, a software engineer, was busy deploying digital solutions for infection control, nursing and midwifery and clinical governance across Scotland, Wales and England, but also Cyprus. The lessons learned from his efforts surpass all my readings on digital transformation in healthcare. This book would not have been possible without the lifelong conversations with my parents and siblings. Costa, Angeliki, Theo and Anthe, I dedicate this book to you.

My academic interest in digital transformation in the context of healthcare begun in early 2002 out of discussions with my then PhD supervisor, Michael Barrett, while a PhD student at the Judge Business School, University of Cambridge. My PhD thesis examined the development and implementation of HEALTHnet, a pilot health information infrastructure for the region of Crete in Greece. Since then I have engaged in a number of research projects exploring among others, contracting and outsourcing arrangements between hospitals in the English NHS and technology vendors in the context of the English National Program for IT (NPfIT), telehealth applications in cardiology and ambulatory and emergency response, digitally enabled decision-making in multidisciplinary cancer care teams and more recently explainable AI technologies in evaluating the intubation of patients in intensive care units. I want to thank my academic colleagues and PhD students that have worked with me on these projects, first and foremost, my long-time collaborators Michael Barrett and Eivor Oborn, and my more recent ones, Nikolay Mehandjiev, Gareth Kitchen, and Tiantian Xian.

During these last two decades, I have had a chance to work with a number of people that are simply impossible to name here, but to whom I owe a debt of gratitude for sharing their knowledge and being patient with me during our conversations. These include doctors, nurses, paramedics and administrative personnel across healthcare organizations, but also digital startup entrepreneurs, software engineers and operational personnel from the companies providing the technology. I want to thank, in particular, Mark Ebbens (previously EMEA Command Centre Lead at GE Healthcare), Mark Edell (Operations Director, Synbiotix), John Sainsbury (Innovation Manager at Greater Manchester Mental Health NHS Trust), Caroline Gadd (previously CEO at Holmusk), Peter Fish (CEO, Mendelian), Maria Chatzou (CEO, Lifebit AI), Stephen Critchlow (Founder, CEO and Chair of Wellbeing Team at Evergreen Life, Chair of the NIHR AI in Healthcare Board), Chris Rushworth (Head of Product, Doctor Care Anywhere), Tara Donelly (Founder Digital Care, Ex-Chief Digital Officer, NHS Digital), Jorge Armanet (Entrepeneur, previously Founder and Former CEO of HealthUnlocked), Marcus Robbins (Chief Digital Advisor, Fujitsu) and James Gannon (VP Quality, Trust and Safety, The PharmaLedger Association).

I also want to thank all the participants of the Digital Health Forum,[1] the delegates of the Digital Transformation in Healthcare course[2] and a separate course on Leading Digital in Healthcare offered by Alliance Manchester Business School to the South Tees NHS Foundation Trust. I am indebted to the knowledge of senior practitioners and policy leaders embedded in the digital health ecosystem, including entrepreneurs, venture capitalists, angel investors and academics. Much of the knowledge shared during these engagements has become part of this book.

I also want to thank other academics who have given me feedback on earlier versions of this book, including Geoff Parker, Carmelo Cennamo, Eric Monteiro, Arun Rai, Elena Karahanna and Rajiv Kohli.

In addition, I would like to thank the publishing team at Routledge, Taylor and Francis, whose feedback throughout the whole process from inception of the initial idea to final publication has been invaluable. In particular, I want to thank Russell George and Amy Thompson, who assisted in keeping this project on schedule and to the three anonymous reviewers, whose constructive feedback helped to further improve the book.

And last, but not least, a big thank you to my wife, Angelina, my daughter Sofia and my son, Andreas, for their unfailing love, support and encouragement throughout the time I was writing this book. You mean everything to me.

Panos Constantinides

Notes

1 https://www.cambridgedigitalinnovation.org/dhf
2 https://www.alliancembs.manchester.ac.uk/study/executive-education/short-business-courses/digital-transformation-in-healthcare/

Figures

Tables

Part 1

Setting the Scene

The Healthcare Context

PART 1 sets the scene for the rest of the book, by describing the complexities of the healthcare context and providing a rationale for an ecosystem approach to digital transformation.

In particular, Chapter 1 reviews the major forces disrupting healthcare services including major shocks such as the COVID-19 pandemic, but also more systemic and institutional forces, including the push toward precision or personalized medicine, and recent advances in digital and biotechnologies. Chapter 1 defines key concepts used throughout the book, including *disruption*, *digital transformation*, *digital maturity* and *ecosystems*. This chapter discusses the emergence of multiple ecosystems, both small and large, and involving different ecosystem actors.

Chapter 2 then provides a deep dive into the key challenges faced by healthcare organizations across the world, primarily because of the prevalence of supply-driven forms of organizing healthcare services. It provides examples of both incumbent organizations in the public and private sector, but also new startups and their efforts to manage challenges ranging from the rising costs of healthcare services, to interoperability challenges between diverse technologies, to ethical and regulatory challenges around data governance.

Finally, Chapter 3 describes how organizations can lead change toward achieving higher value for patients. Value is discussed in relation to the healthcare delivery cycle, exploring how different ecosystem actors get involved in this cycle's distinct processes, going beyond healthcare service providers, to also examine the role of medical device manufacturers, diagnostic centers, biotech and pharmaceutical companies and digital service integrators, among others. Following this discussion, the focus shifts to how each of these ecosystem actors can develop unique value propositions by leveraging digital technologies. Chapter 3 outlines different levels of digital maturity, offering a blueprint by which healthcare organizations can identify where they stand and how they can begin to digitally transform themselves.

DOI: 10.4324/9781032619569-1

1 Disruption and Digital Transformation in Healthcare

Disruption and digital transformation have received great attention in recent years, both in the popular press and in professional and industry reports. The primary focus has been on the unique capabilities offered by new digital technologies such as blockchain, Artificial Intelligence (AI), the Internet of Things (IoT) and cloud computing and the ways by which these can now be accessed on-demand through various devices. Digital technologies may generate disruption and an urgency for digital transformation, but they are not the only drivers for transforming healthcare. Disruptive events like the COVID-19 pandemic, the shift toward personalized medicine and the empowerment of patients, as well as changes in competitive dynamics between incumbent organizations and new startups are generating not only new demands from patients and healthcare professionals but also new supply dynamics from various ecosystem actors. Together, these systemic drivers act as disruptive forces in the digital transformation of healthcare.

This chapter introduces disruption and digital transformation and discusses how they impact the delivery of healthcare services. It discusses how individual organizations in healthcare are faced with an increasing complexity due to limited resources, infrastructure and skills, as well as institutional and regulatory pressures to transform services in order to meet patient demands. No single organization can navigate the complexity of the healthcare landscape on its own. The chapter elaborates on how complexity can be reduced and risks can be mitigated if organizations take part in healthcare ecosystems where they can synergistically combine resources and capabilities with others. Organizations can learn to leverage new digital technologies and respond to disruption through ecosystems. This forms the key thesis of the book.

1.1 COVID-19: The Ultimate Disruption

The COVID-19 pandemic has disrupted global healthcare systems and has accelerated digital transformation.[1] It has brought to the surface long-standing digital and health inequalities and has pushed for changes that in normal times could have taken years to implement, but were instead made in a matter of hours. The risks of doing nothing were bigger in light of the uncertainty surrounding the pandemic.

The COVID-19 pandemic has exposed many vulnerabilities in healthcare systems globally[2]; it has caused the shortage of testing, personal protective equipment (PPE) and ventilators, especially in India[3]; it has disproportionally affected marginalized segments of the population[4]; it has led to a shortage of healthcare workers and limited to no access to vaccines[5]; and has adversely impacted the global supply chain.[6] In the European Union, the COVID-19 pandemic has fueled large-scale experimentation ranging from

DOI: 10.4324/9781032619569-2

failed attempts at building herd immunity,[7] to varied approaches in applying lockdowns and social distancing, to distributing and using PPE and life support medical devices, as well as implementing phased vaccination programs.[8] During the pandemic, hospitals and primary care centers across different countries have also faced significant financial challenges. For example, hospitals in the USA were losing $1.4 billion a day. A 2020 survey carried out by the American Hospital Association[9] found that inpatient volumes dropped to 19 percent, whereas outpatient volumes dropped to 34 percent. And this while expenses for tests, PPE and other consumables went up by $3.8 billion. The year 2020 alone had losses of $323 billion. While there was provider relief and federal funding, that only covered about 50–60 percent of these losses. This led to furloughs and layoffs of staff[11] and other very difficult decisions such as shutting down or limiting volumes of services delivered. Some hospitals had to eliminate elective surgeries altogether and to focus only on critical care.[12] Nurses who had previously been assigned other roles were retrained to be able to do critical care,[13] and admin and support personnel were shifted across healthcare systems with an emphasis on eliminating excess capacity and duplication of services.

Public health surveillance and real-time patient safety were also impacted with new technologies and health prevention practices. Public health surveillance is the "ongoing systematic collection, analysis, and interpretation of health-related data essential to planning, implementation, and evaluation of public health practice", including the "timely dissemination of these data to those responsible for prevention and control".[14] Various track and trace mobile apps[15] have been developed during the COVID-19 pandemic forming an active surveillance system for COVID-19 infections. Contact tracing and tracking is a highly effective active surveillance system that has been a cornerstone of containing infectious disease outbreaks in the past, from HIV to influenza. However, as evidence from the COVID-19 outbreak has shown, we lack testing resources and coordinated procedures across regions, states and international organizations, to render contact tracing a viable method of population-level transmission mitigation.[16] Also, evidence has shown that COVID-19 had both a long period of infectiousness and a pre-symptomatic and asymptomatic spread.[17] This made contact tracing difficult because its success relied on individuals' ability to recall contacts while contagious including prior to feeling ill. Finally, while evidence suggests contact tracing and associated quarantine policies do not require 100 percent compliance to be effective, compliance has presented inequitable burden to individuals and under-resourced communities.[18] As the example of COVID-19 indicates, active surveillance systems are resource intensive and not always effective – even though current advances in mobile app tracking and tracing have significantly improved public health surveillance. For example, a study of the impact of the NHS COVID-19 app for England and Wales, from its launch on 24 September 2020 through to the end of December 2020, estimated that a 30 percent app uptake averted approximately one for every four infections.[19]

The biggest challenges faced by public health surveillance systems relate not only to abilities to integrate data collection and data analytics capabilities through common interfaces but also to build the necessary skill set within healthcare organizations to be able to interpret public health data. Underlying this challenge is the ability to coordinate efforts across disparate communities and regions,[20] across healthcare organizations with variable resources and most importantly to generate data and health prevention practices that will be relevant to individuals, not just populations. Studies examining the value of achieving such universal coordination on public health surveillance among healthcare systems and healthcare providers have shown that the relation of input epidemiological data to output health outcomes is questionable, given the uneven public health characteristics of different countries[21] and the varied practices in public health reporting. The costs of achieving such universal coordination are very high, while the benefits for individual patients are unclear.[22]

At the same time, the COVID-19 pandemic has accelerated the adoption of mobile technologies that generated increased benefits for individual patients. Telemedicine, in all its incarnations over the last 40 years or so, has been constrained by legacy regulation, non-interoperability between systems and barriers to data exchange.[23] Within a very short period, technical and non-technical barriers have been removed when it became clear that telemedicine enabled many doctors to continue to care safely for their patients remotely while avoiding risks of virus transmission.

The number of health apps on the two leading digital platforms (iOS and Android) has more than doubled in the last few years. This rise is being driven by the increasing ownership of smartphones, as well as improved connectivity across different parts of the world. In addition to this, the COVID-19 pandemic has dramatically reshaped consumer habits with smartphones and mobile apps becoming central to our lives. According to AppAnnie,[24] health and fitness apps have set global records for the highest level of both weekly downloads and consumer spend at 59 million and $36 million, respectively, during the first month of the pandemic, in March 2020 – a growth of 40 percent and 10 percent from the weekly average of January and February 2020. In addition, medical apps have experienced an acceleration of 65 percent in downloads globally during the pandemic, pointing to an increased reliance and escalation of consumer trust in these apps in contrast to face-to-face consultations with their doctors.[25] There has been a significant growth in downloads for popular platforms, including Telehealth by SimplePractice, Doccla, Doctor on Demand, Doctor Care Anywhere and Doximity. For example, these apps reported significant increases in daily virtual medical visits during the pandemic across regions compared to the expected number of visits based on historical patterns.

This growth in the use of telehealth has correlated with the movement and impact of the virus. These trends have been more profound in Asia, with South Korea and India experiencing the highest growth in medical app downloads during the pandemic at 135 percent from January to February 2020 and 90 percent growth from January to April 2020, respectively. In South Korea, the top two medical apps that saw the largest growth in downloads were coronavirus tracking apps. In India, Medlife, Netmeds and Practo were the top three medical apps by growth in downloads, respectively, during this time. Medlife and Netmeds offer delivery of medical prescriptions and Practo facilitates telehealth consultations with doctors. All three apps are examples of demand for socially distanced medical services. In a recent survey by Black Book Market Research,[26] 59 percent of patients reported that they were more likely to use telehealth services due to the ongoing pandemic, and almost half of physicians leveraged telehealth services as the COVID-19 pandemic continued to disrupt normal operations.[27] While telehealth has played a significant role during the pandemic, its adoption by both patients and healthcare professionals has continued to accelerate after the pandemic and will influence continued digital transformation.

The COVID-19 pandemic has broken down the competitive barriers between traditional providers and digital healthcare delivery companies. For example, digital first companies such as Teladoc[28] and Doctor Care Anywhere[29] are gaining traction with national payers and private insurance providers in the UK and US to provide subscriptions to different services, primarily in primary care. The same is true for Ping An Good Doctor in China.[30] Interestingly, Ping An started connecting healthcare providers and patients through health insurance before eventually enabling doctors external to affiliated providers to consult patients remotely, offering a wide range of virtual health services. They more recently provided application programming interfaces (API) to third-party developers to add complementary services for providers, doctors and patients, including applications for AI-enabled radiology and pathology, as well as mobile payments. Ping An Good Doctor is China's largest digital healthcare platform, with more than 200 million users and collaborating with over 3,000 hospitals to provide services such as hospital referrals, appointments and inpatient arrangements. It also partners with more than 2,000 healthcare institutions, including physical examination centers, dental clinics, cosmetic surgery institutions and more than 15,000 pharmacy outlets to provide personalized health and wellness services to their users. Ping An Health is an example of a growing healthcare ecosystem involving various ecosystem actors, including payers, healthcare providers, medical device manufacturers and pharmaceutical and biotech organizations. The COVID-19 pandemic has laid the ground for a new normal in healthcare services, one that is bound to be transformed by new digital technologies and spanning organizational boundaries.

1.2 Disruptive Changes in Healthcare Services and the Role of the Empowered Patient

Disruption, of course, is not just caused from such disruptive events as the COVID-19 pandemic. Disruption is also caused from institutional and competitive pressures from various ecosystem actors toward digital transformation.

In the last two decades or so, there has been increasing pressure toward personalized or precision medicine from healthcare providers, doctors, patients and even payers.[31] These pressures have been institutionalized in new policies and have had ripple effects across other ecosystem actors such as pharmaceutical and biotech organizations as well as medical device manufacturers.[32] Personalized medicine is the targeted process of administering the most appropriate treatment for an individual patient at the most appropriate time and with the correct dose. Others have extended this notion of precision medicine as the need to shift our mindset to a focus on *preventing disease*[33] as opposed to simply treating disease. The key objective is to handle each patient as a unique individual away from the current one-size-fits-all trial-and-error approach that characterizes most healthcare practices today. Personalized medicine uses molecular diagnostic tools to identify specific biological markers, including genetic and physiological, to help assess methods of preventing disease as opposed to treating it after the fact. By combining the data from these tests with a patient's medical history and personal circumstances, healthcare providers can develop targeted prevention plans first and foremost. This goal toward preventing disease is also linked to continued efforts by healthcare systems around the globe to have zero patient encounters – to avoid expensive diagnostic and treatment practices in hospitals.[34] The use of wearables, home monitoring and other sensor technologies aims to achieve this goal and feeds into the need toward personalized medicine. Patients want to be able to manage their own health records to monitor their health and wellness, on demand, at the comfort of their own home with smart technologies, as in the example of the Evergreen Life App[10].

First, there is demand for safer and more effective treatment options. To give an example, data has shown that major drugs such as hypertension drugs like ACE and heart failure drugs such as beta blockers have varied effectiveness across different patients, while the side effects also vary.[35] If we extrapolate for those inefficiencies where drugs do not work to the cost of ineffectiveness to the healthcare system, a lot of money could be saved and reinvested in more targeted prevention and treatment plans. In fact, ineffective therapies can cause harmful side effects that can further increase the costs to the healthcare system. Some studies have shown that between 7 and 15 percent of hospital admissions are linked to adverse drug reactions.[36] There are hundreds of thousands of deaths per year from such adverse drug reactions,[37] and many patients experience adverse drug reactions during hospital stay. Thus, both the financial costs and the cost of human lives are high when following more traditional, population-level health prevention and treatment plans where the focus is on how specific treatments work on average across a population segment. Clinical trials on effective drug treatments "take heterogeneous inputs (the people in the study or studies) and come up with homogeneous results (the average result across all those people). Evidence-based medicine then insists that we apply those average findings back to individuals. The problem is that no patient is strictly average".[38] In contrast, precision medicine can provide more tailored, personalized healthcare plans, especially in the case of chronic conditions, as well as conditions based on genetic markers. The key objective is to assess the risk of following plan A as opposed to plan B not for the average individual in the population segment, but rather in relation to the unique mix of symptoms and risk factors for a specific patient. Such a personalized approach would weigh the risk versus reward versus cost of therapy for individual patients while paying more attention to maintaining the quality of life for a longer period of time.

Second, personalized medicine is driven by recent advances in biotechnologies, especially whole genome sequencing. Whole genome sequencing offers the ability to identify rare variants in genetic disorders, enabling a better understanding and management of rare and chronic diseases.[39] The first sequence of the human genome was completed in 2003 and cost approximately $150 million.[40] Since then, the cost of whole genome sequencing has dropped from $14,000 in 2006 to $1,000 in 2015. Today the cost is somewhere in between $500 and 1,000.[41] This drop in cost is closely aligned with faster computing processors, improved data storage and nanotechnology, as well as advancements in genomics and molecular technologies. But it is not just the cost that has dropped; it is also the speed by which human genome sequencing can be done. From a timeline of 6–8 years, some companies like Illumina[42] are now able to do multiple whole genome sequences in a day. And finally, from big laboratories where human genome sequencing could previously be done, we are now in an era where portable devices are used to do the genome sequencing.[43] Whole genome sequencing is a disruptive technology that is further driving transformation toward personalized medicine. Whole genome sequencing can help explain how patients with the same disease exhibit different medical trajectories, while reacting differently to treatment plans. Although all human beings are 99.8 percent identical, we each have about three to five million differences in our genome compared to another person. Certainly, most of those differences are common variants and exist in a few percent in the population. Only a very small fraction of those variants is relatively rare. Whole genome sequencing enables the identification of the risks involved for getting a disease if a variant is present, as well as which of those variants may protect us from getting the disease.

In the UK, the 100,000 Genomes Project[44] sequenced the genomes of 100,000 individuals affected by a rare disease or cancer. Approximately 6–7 percent of the UK population is affected by cancer or a rare disease each year. Cancer begins because of changes in genes within what was a normal cell. Although a cancer starts with the same DNA as the patient, it develops mutations or changes which enable the tumor to grow and spread. By taking DNA from the tumor and DNA from the patient's normal cells and comparing them, the 100,000 Genomes Project was able to detect the precise changes in a patient's cells. This pilot project has now been transformed to routine genomics services on rare and chronic diseases provided by Genomics England,[45] a wholly owned subsidiary of the Department of Health and Social Care. Knowing and understanding these changes strongly indicates which treatments will be the most effective. Genomics has already started to guide and inform doctors about the best treatment for individual patients or their relatives. Knowledge of the whole genome sequencing may identify the cause of chronic and rare diseases and help point the way to new methods of preventing these diseases, as well as learning to live with them while managing the risks involved. As most rare diseases are inherited, the genomes of the affected individual (usually a child) plus two of their closest blood relatives are included to pinpoint the cause of the condition. Acting early to identify the genomic and biological markers of a disease – as early as birth – can help an individual prevent disease. Changing nutritional and exercise patterns on the basis of genomic and biological markers can help individuals avoid the onset of negative consequences such as falling victims of the metabolic syndrome that can spiral genetic disease out of control much earlier than otherwise.[46]

Beyond national initiatives like the 100,000 Genomes Project, there are also many private initiatives. One example is Human Longevity, a facility that enables individuals to have their genome sequenced, to then predict the probability that they will develop a disease or to suffer from a medical condition such as heart failure in the future. Human Longevity combines a large database of genomic and phenotypic data with imaging data and machine learning to drive discoveries and deliver curated personal health information. The scientists at Human Longevity published the results of a three-year study[47] that enrolled 1,190 presumed healthy participants aged 18 and above. To the surprise of the participants, 86 percent of them were found to be genetic carriers of recessive diseases such as Alzheimer's and 24 percent of them were found to have a rare genetic mutation that will affect their health in the future. A total of 206 unique medically significant variants in 111 genes were identified. These are shocking findings with potentially life-changing outcomes, especially for the higher risk participants. After this study, these higher risk participants were recommended to undergo additional tests and enroll in preventative measures to manage their health risk.

Third, whole genome sequencing, together with other technologies such as medical imaging, biosensors and machine learning algorithms that detect patterns in the data, is significantly augmenting medical decision-making, while empowering patients to take a more active role in the management of their health and wellness. Empowered patients engage in preventive health activities and self-management of their genetic and biological propensity to develop a disease. Such engagement ranges from monitoring blood glucose levels with small, portable devices[48] to the use of full-body, comprehensive physical, mental and emotional self-tracking technologies.[49] The key objective of patient empowerment is the right and responsibility of patients to access health information and make their own health-related decisions using their own data.[50] This is an extension of precision and personalized medicine, whereby patients are not just receivers of data and knowledge by their carers, but rather they become actively engaged in the production, analysis and interpretation of such data and knowledge. The pursuit of quantifying one's self can have several benefits including learning how to live with a disease while improving one's understanding of how to make behavioral changes that can improve their physical, mental and emotional health. Research has shown that self-tracking technologies are widely used in people's daily lives and healthcare to promote health and well-being.[51]

However, there are also risks associated with quantified self projects. Some critics argue that the use of self-tracking devices can promote extreme forms of healthism and individualism.[52] For example, the billionaire entrepreneur Bryan Johnson has developed a so-called blueprint[53] with a team of 30 doctors to improve his physical and mental performance. According to his website, he spent two years and millions of dollars developing an algorithm that takes better care of him than he can himself. The blueprint incorporates not just a daily nutrition and supplement routine but also a series of weekly and monthly tests, including ultrasounds, colonoscopies, MRI scans and blood tests to empower him to make better decisions about his health and well-being. However, some critics have raised concerns not only about the extreme measures taken by Johnson and the potential risks associated with such an approach, including the high costs of following the blueprint, but also the potential for harm from unproven treatments and the ethical implications of such extreme measures.[54] Some have argued that the techno-utopian discourses concerning the possibilities afforded by self-tracking technologies do not acknowledge the complexities and ambivalences that are part of self-monitoring health, for both patients and healthcare providers. These include "the emotions and resistances they provoke, their contribution to the burden of self-care and the invisible work on the part of healthcare workers that they require to operate".[55] Empowerment should be understood as both a process and an outcome,[56] and it involves a patient's interaction not only with other patients suffering from similar conditions but also with doctors and other ecosystem actors.

Indeed, patient empowerment has disrupted the role of many ecosystem actors in healthcare service provision and management. It has put more pressure on healthcare providers such as hospitals and their specialized experts including doctors to become more digitally augmented. Doctors are no longer practicing medicine; they have become part of a team of multidisciplinary experts including data scientists, molecular biologists and technology engineers. This team has greater expertise to implement more targeted plans for personalized medicine in comparison to single doctors without digital technologies. Together with this multidisciplinary team, doctors are in a better position to make informed decisions about how patients should interpret data about their disease. This is paramount in avoiding some of the risks mentioned above in relation to self-tracking devices for better monitoring one's health. These technologies are important and critical for helping patients – especially those suffering from chronic diseases – to receive remote, on-demand care round the clock. However, to achieve this, doctors and other carers need to be trained on how to use those technologies themselves, as well as to be supported by technology experts that can help them interpret data generated from those technologies. Overall, the move toward preventive, personalized medicine has generated not only new challenges but also transformative opportunities on healthcare ecosystems.

1.3 Digital Technology as a Transformative Force

Based on the discussion so far, we can define **disruption** as *a disturbance to the status quo that can create significant uncertainty about how to respond and adjust.*

Disruption can be caused by major shocks[57] such as the COVID-19 pandemic, but it can also be caused by gradual institutional and competitive pressures from various ecosystem actors toward change. Institutional pressures emerge from an understanding that current practices are ineffective, unsustainable and potentially posing risks to health outcomes as well as the financial viability of organizations within healthcare ecosystems. Competitive pressures emerge from new advances in medical knowledge as caused by new technologies such as whole genome sequencing. New ecosystem actors can leverage these new technologies to disrupt the dominance of incumbent actors while at the same time transforming existing practices.

According to disruptive innovation theory,[58] by and large, a disruptive technology is initially embraced by the least profitable customers in a market. Hence, most companies with a practiced discipline of listening to their best customers and identifying new products that promise greater profitability and growth are rarely able to build a case for investing in disruptive technologies until it is too late. Disruption through such competitive dynamics is generally perceived from the perspective of organizations that are heavily invested in old ways of doing things and whose typical or planned course of development is interrupted. As the proliferation of new business processes and technologies leads to change in established industry structures, organizations face severe pressure to respond. Such responses can prompt fundamental transformation to operations, the legacy technologies and routine practices and even the identities of the organizations and professionals within them.

In more recent years, the threat of digital disruption has increased through a shift in the focus on supply-side operations to provide healthcare services to patients to demand-side pressures from empowered patients for more on-demand services, often delivered through digital platforms,[59] as discussed in the previous sections. Patients seek and access healthcare service through such digital platforms as Doccla, Doctor Care Anywhere and Teladoc; they use personal devices for healthcare monitoring and interact with different ecosystem actors on demand. This means that there are now different interdependencies between ecosystem actors. The interdependencies between them are not always based on competition, as past theories of disruptive innovation have supported. Rather, ecosystem interdependencies are now based on complementary resources and capabilities.[60]

For example, Pfizer, a big incumbent pharmaceutical company, partnered with a small biotechnology company, BioNTech, to leverage the latter's mRNA technology capabilities and speed up the process of clinical and research activities toward providing a COVID-19 vaccine much faster than other incumbent pharmaceutical and biotech companies. BioNTech has more recently partnered with InstaDeep to generate insights from public and proprietary data using machine learning capabilities to identify novel biological targets and predictive markers.[61] Together with Pfizer and InstaDeep, BioNTech also aims to optimize drug manufacturing and supply chain capabilities, thus slowly expanding their ecosystem. Like BioNTech, Moderna has opened their mRNA technology to other pharmaceutical companies in areas including immuno-oncology, viral vaccines and therapies for rare diseases.[62] These strategic moves have generated new complementary resources and capabilities spanning new ecosystems. Complementary resources and capabilities,[63] such as the machine learning capabilities of a new digital startup and the data resources of a large hospital, can be synergistically combined. Through such synergistic combination, diverse actors can fill in gaps in their internal knowledge and competences and respond to disruption, while also opening opportunities for innovation and value cocreation.

Accordingly, **digital transformation** can be understood as *the ongoing process of responding to disruption by using digital technologies to synergistically combine resources and capabilities for value creation.* Digital transformation is not a one-off project; it is ongoing since disruption is also continuous. As previously discussed, disruption may be radical and acute, like the COVID-19 pandemic, but it may also be gradual and chronically infused through institutional pressures to transform healthcare services.

Like technological transformations of the past, digital transformation is tightly interwoven with both physical (e.g., MRI scanners) and digital technologies (e.g., machine learning algorithms). Like earlier technology, digital technology is modular, enabling it to be decomposed into smaller components or aggregated into larger infrastructures.[64] Decomposition and aggregation relationships between digital technologies offer ways to reduce complexity and increase flexibility with the help of standardized interfaces.[65] Standardized interfaces capture each modular component's implementation details while at the same time enabling interdependencies between them. In this way, digital technologies can be developed as bundled products such as enterprise resource planning systems. However, whereas non-digital technologies are nested and fixed to a product hierarchy, digital technologies can be product agnostic, modular and generative.[66]

Product agnosticism differentiates digital technologies from non-digital technologies. A software application or a machine learning algorithm can be embedded in multiple devices, from a smartphone to an MRI scanner and an operating theater or a ward (via IoT sensors). This contrasts with conventional technologies such as a microscope or an X-ray imaging system that is nested and fixed within the same product hierarchy. For example, the components that make up an X-ray imaging system cannot be used to build a microscope and vice versa. In contrast, the product agnosticism of digital technologies allows them to be easily combined to perform a wide variety of functions across devices from different product hierarchies.

Modularity enables digital technologies to be composed of distinct and relatively self-sufficient units loosely coupled through well-defined interfaces.[67] Modularity makes technologies easier to change. Various modules of digital technologies can thus be readily recombined to generate systems with new functionalities.[68] Electronic patient records can be linked with machine learning applications in ward management, diagnostics and drug discovery. These applications can then be used as modular components that feed into services offered by many different organizations from hospitals, to insurers, biotech and research through standardized interfaces such as API. These applications can be accessible in wearables, mobile devices and IoT sensors in buildings and even human bodies.

The product agnosticism and modularity of digital technology create a generative combination of capabilities and resources between seemingly disparate actors. Digital technology can entail contributions by heterogeneous complementors that can constantly bring about new value propositions to healthcare ecosystems.

At the same time, the product agnosticism and modularity of digital technologies raise the level of technical complexity, the tacit knowledge and expertise involved, as well as the risks underlying the development and implementation of new technology combinations. Organizations will exhibit varying levels of digital maturity, and this affects their readiness to respond to disruption and digitally transform.

Digital maturity is the *measure of an organization's capabilities to create and capture value by leveraging digital technologies.* While some organizations may exhibit high capabilities in clinical skills and resources such as robotic surgery, others may exhibit high capabilities in data analytics and computing resources. Others may exhibit low capabilities in all of the above. More importantly, for each of these capabilities, organizations need to establish appropriate governance rules to be able to create and capture value with digital technologies.[69]

1.4   The Need for an Ecosystem Approach: Combining Capabilities and Resources for Multilateral Value Cocreation

The discussion so far may give the impression that the book places sole emphasis on developed economies where most research and development in new technological solutions is taking place. After all, which parts of the world have access to large computing facilities, data storage and network architectures with high bandwidth connections? Which parts of the world benefit from access to secondary, tertiary and even specialized healthcare services and treatment such as whole genome sequencing and mRNA vaccinations against cancer? Which countries have university hospitals and other digitally mature healthcare organizations that can deploy such cutting-edge technologies? The answer is developed economies in the UK, the European Union, the USA and China, among others.

However, this does not mean that these same developed economies do not include healthcare organizations with low digital maturity that suffer from the same challenges as those in developing economies. In England, hospitals are under an "impending crisis, with capital restrictions limiting investment in buildings, infrastructure and equipment" that impact the quality and safety of care.[70] The USA is also suffering from similar issues.[71] No country is immune to disruption, and certainly no single organization can navigate the complexity of the healthcare landscape on its own. By extension, no individual organization can take on the task of digital transformation by itself. Complexity can be reduced, and risks can be mitigated if organizations can synergistically combine complementary resources and capabilities across healthcare ecosystems.

An **ecosystem** is *an organizational form that is less hierarchical than firms and yet more centrally governed than traditional markets.*[72] In an ecosystem, interdependent actors form multilateral partnerships to create and capture value.

An ecosystem is composed of multiple, heterogeneous actors, whose partnerships are co-dependent. Ecosystem actors are dependent on one another for capabilities and resources they do not have but which are necessary for a joint value proposition to emerge. This set of actors can synergistically combine capabilities and resources to create value propositions that are not hierarchically controlled by a single actor, as in the case of supply chain networks. That is, ecosystem actors can retain some control and claims over their resources and capabilities. Although some ecosystem actors will be more digitally mature than others, something that would place them in a position to orchestrate the ecosystem, no actor can unilaterally set the terms for the types, prices and quantities of the capabilities produced. None of these decisions are hierarchically controlled, although an ecosystem orchestrator can define the technology standards and governance rules (e.g., revenue share models, access to resources) upon which capabilities can be produced and value created and captured.

For example, an ecosystem can emerge between medical device manufacturers that coordinate with digital service providers to offer seamless access to electronic health records within healthcare organizations; biodata banks, machine learning experts and omics analysis experts that coordinate to offer data analytics capabilities of different types of data; healthcare service providers and insurance companies that coordinate to offer healthcare services according to different payment plans; and pharmaceutical and biotech companies that coordinate to offer clinical trial and drug development capabilities. Together these sets of complementors can contribute to the ecosystem's joint value proposition to serve a patient population. One group of resources and capabilities offered by one complementor set depends on another complementor set to realize the joint value proposition. Such joint value propositions can increase value creation and value capture for all ecosystem actors as the value of one set of resources and capabilities increases when combined with others, as seen in Figure 1.1.

What differentiates ecosystems from supplier-mediated arrangements (including those organized through a system or service integrator) is that, in ecosystems, end-users, such as patients, can choose among the capabilities and resources that are provided by each ecosystem actor and can also, in some cases, choose how they are combined. For example, a patient can choose the core services of a primary care provider, but then they can decide which specialized services (e.g., mental health services) to buy and from which provider, instead of buying a combined product or service by a single primary care provider. Virtual care platforms like Doccla[73] are an example of such primary care service.

In the example shown in Figure 1.1, a healthcare organization such as a large teaching hospital can act as the ecosystem orchestrator by defining the governance structures upon which different ecosystem actors can synergistically combine their capabilities. Thus, ecosystems can span more widely than a single hospital (i.e., an organizational hierarchy) but narrower than an open marketplace, by bringing together a curated set of complementors through common technological standards and governance rules. This is a curated set of complementors in that, although anyone can participate, those that do, have to follow the technological standards and governance rules that are defined by the orchestrator. This is what differentiates ecosystems from open marketplaces.

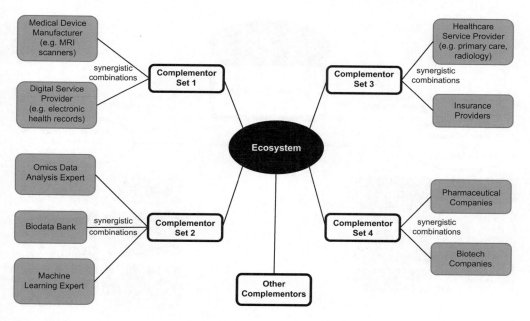

Figure 1.1 Synergistic Combinations in an Ecosystem.

Digital platforms play a key technological role in the orchestration process. A **digital platform** *provides a set of technological resources (including interfaces, development tools and infrastructures) to enable value-creating interactions between producers and consumers of digital services in an ecosystem.*[74]

Thus, by deploying a digital platform, a healthcare organization can orchestrate synergistic combinations of services, while offering patients a choice as to who to buy those services from. In contrast, without such a digital platform and the ecosystem supported by it, a patient would have to buy a combined product or service by the healthcare organization, without ever interacting with, or knowing about, those individual complementors. A healthcare organization would be acting as a service integrator in such a case, as patients would never have direct interaction with the complementors. Instead, in a digital platform ecosystem, different ecosystem actors can directly interact.

As seen in Figure 1.2, there are three sets of actors in a digital platform ecosystem. First, the ecosystem orchestrator is the organization responsible for providing the technological platform and setting the governance rules through which ecosystem participants will interact. The second set of actors is complementors who are the producers of services and products. These may vary from software, machine learning and other technology providers, but could also include biodata banks, research institutes and even independent healthcare providers. For example, doctors on platforms such as Babylon Health and Doximity could be considered complementors as they are contracted to offer services on demand to other ecosystem actors, including patients but potentially also to other healthcare service providers. Thus, the third set of actors, namely, the users, could include not only patients but also other ecosystem actors that consume services and products. So, for instance, a hospital can consume not only services provided by technology providers but also services provided by other healthcare providers. For example,

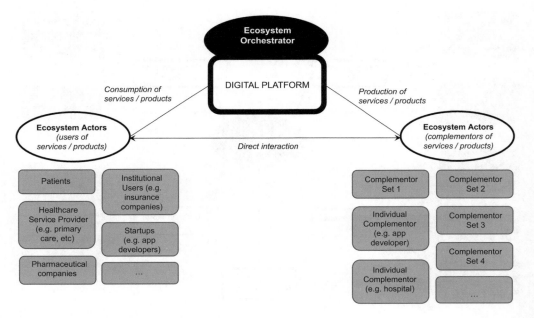

Figure 1.2 A Digital Platform Ecosystem.

a hospital with no resident radiologists can consume radiology services provided by another hospital that has extra capacity.

Ecosystems have different degrees of scale, from smaller ones orchestrated by a healthcare organization to larger ones orchestrated by big tech companies like Amazon. A large ecosystem like Amazon's Web Services (AWS) for Health[75] can orchestrate a wider set of complementors for a wider set of customers. Amazon's AWS for Health provides on-demand cloud computing services via a common technological infrastructure to different organizations, in many cases to enable these organizations to provide digital services to their own customers. Amazon orchestrates the ecosystem by enabling different organizations to select software produced not only by Amazon but also by providers including Couchbase, IBM, Microsoft, Red Hat and SAP, as well as many widely used open-source products, including Wordpress and MediaWiki. The AWS ecosystem includes many third-party healthcare software, machine learning models, services and even data that can serve biotech organizations, medical device manufacturers, payers and healthcare providers with varied pricing models.[76] A digital platform ecosystem of this scale can provide the necessary incentives – in the form of technology solutions, knowledge and data exchange, as well as monetary rewards – that can attract different ecosystem actors, with each of those acting as complementors for one another.

In an ecosystem, all actors can potentially produce and consume services and products. All actors can participate in value creation and value capture. This is a unique differentiator from more conventional approaches to digital transformation whereby organizations either create value for, or receive value from, other organizations. For example, a hospital purchases a new system for managing electronic patient records from a technology vendor. The technology vendor creates value for the hospital that receives the system. This is referred to as *"value-in-exchange"*, whereby a vendor sells a product to a customer and captures value from the transaction.[77] This value exchange is a one-off transaction with neither party engaged in repeated interactions toward further value creation. In contrast, when there are co-dependencies between ecosystem actors, then the roles of user and complementor are interchangeable; both create and receive value from one another. In this case, there is *"value-in-use"*.[78] Value is no longer a one-off transaction, but rather a continued process, whereby all ecosystem actors can both produce and consume services and products. In the Amazon's AWS for Health, for example, healthcare service providers are not just consumers of services. Their use of AWS complements produces troves of clinical and other types of data that feed into yet new services and products, attracting yet new third-party complementors in a virtuous cycle of value cocreation.

No single ecosystem actor can address the range of patient needs, nor can they solely manage the ways in which patients engage with different modalities of healthcare services from pharmacy, primary and tertiary care, as well as diagnostic and support services for chronic and other conditions. It requires distinct capabilities and resources to provide such services, while at the same time expanding to new modalities of digital care including home and self-care through patient engagement and remote monitoring. Equally, distinct capabilities are needed to provide access to social and community networks related to a patient's holistic health, as well as to monitor daily life activities, including fitness, wellness and nutrition. Finally, managing payments, insurance claims and providing financial support including operations require yet other distinct capabilities and resources. Such capabilities and resources need to be synergistically combined to provide the necessary conditions and incentives for value creation and capture for ecosystem actors.

Increasingly, patients expect and demand services to be delivered to them on their personal devices, including smartphones, smart watches and other wearables. Patients can log in on Babylon Health, for example, to get their symptoms checked by the AI-enabled symptom checker,[79] before booking virtual consultations with a primary care doctor. During the COVID-19 pandemic, if their primary care doctor found that these patients experienced early symptoms of the COVID-19 virus, they were in a position to recommend that they have a rapid lateral flow test as a first action. The patient was able to order a test kit online such as Randox,[80] have it delivered at their home address and do the test by themselves. They could also download an app such as the Randox Certifly[81] and have the app scan the QR code of the test and carry an image analysis of the test result. All the above points of service were offered without the patient ever leaving their home. All were within reach of their personal smartphone.

Certainly, all these services require various ecosystem actors to coordinate before the services are seamlessly delivered to the patient. For example, Babylon Health needs to onboard and coordinate individual primary care doctors. Primary care doctors in the National Health Service (NHS) in England are paid based on the number of patients on their list.[82] Indeed, this is true for most national health systems around the world. However, the number of patients on a primary care doctor's list is very much dependent on geographical location and proximity. Babylon Health and other such digital platforms allow primary care doctors to expand their geographical boundaries and scale up the number of patients they cater for. But it is not just about financial incentives. It is also about flexibility and managing the work–life balance for primary care doctors, who just like patients can also attend to their personal and work needs via their personal smartphone device. By enabling patients and primary care doctors to interact digitally and on-demand, such digital platforms give a choice to both. This choice is informed based on feedback and recommendations from previous interactions. Together with the AI symptom checker, primary care doctors offer on-demand, remote primary care services to patients.

Ecosystem capabilities expand beyond primary care doctors and their patients. Through digital platforms, employers can receive invaluable insights on the health of their employees so that they can make informed decisions regarding health insurance and well-being planning.[83] Indeed, national payers, employers and insurers use such digital platforms to provide incentives for prevention of disease and healthy lifestyles while offering different opportunities for lowering claims costs. Ping An, Tencent and Alibaba in China have been able to scale affordable health services and tie those to a wide variety of health insurance packages based on patient needs in an unprecedented way.[84] All these ecosystem actors depend on digital technology providers, including cloud storage for electronic health records and blockchain for managing financial transactions securely. For example, Alibaba Cloud is the biggest cloud service provider in China, and together with its data intelligence technologies it is helping several healthcare service providers optimize a wide variety of services.[85] Moreover, Ping An uses OneChain, a proprietary technology that can process over 100,000 transactions per second in a highly secure way, across Ping An's ecosystem.[86]

These digital platform ecosystems are very much defined by the needs of different patient populations, but are, at the same time, augmented by the synergistic combinations of resources – in particular, digital data – and capabilities between ecosystem actors. On the one hand, healthy patients who are keen to monitor their own health and fitness often set personal wellness goals and have higher expectations on digital touchpoints with access to different modalities of care.[87] These patients demand constant insights from their data toward more personalized care. On the other hand, patients with multiple, complex chronic conditions will require more creative solutions that involve both physical and digital touchpoints. For these patients, coordination between ecosystem actors will have to ensure that a team of carers – from family members, social carers and medical staff – is augmented with digital technologies to be able to deliver both digital and in-person services, at home or near the home.[88] Along these two extremes, there will be multiple other patient segments with various needs that need to be digitally supported. The key is in addressing the needs of each of these segments while offering personalized services to individual patients and reducing the complexity behind their access to different modalities of care. The patient-oriented nature of these digital platform ecosystems aims to increase the number of digital touchpoints, with the goal of modifying patient behavior and improving outcomes.

Despite the opportunities to transform patient outcomes, while scaling service provision through ecosystems, many organizations, from providers such as primary, secondary and tertiary care, as well as payers, such as the state or private insurers, have not yet clearly articulated their ecosystem strategy. Many of these organizations are not able to orchestrate ecosystems because they lack the necessary capabilities and resources – human, technological, operational and financial – and are also faced with several constraints, from legacy systems and unclear data strategies. Many of these organizations also have poor digital transformation strategies in place that take into account the training and skill development needed to augment their workforce. All is not lost, however, as organizations can partner with digital technology providers on new and emerging ecosystems, while focusing on their core value propositions.

Payers, for example, have access to many different ecosystem actors, while being able to shape regulation in a highly regulated sector. They can influence the purchase of digitally enabled healthcare services from pre- and post-acute care delivery systems. Their core value proposition can be attractive to digital technology providers like Amazon, Google and Microsoft. These technology providers already have the set of technology resources and capabilities to orchestrate digitally enabled healthcare services across modalities of care. For example, Amazon already offers primary and other types of care to its employees and has the cloud infrastructure as well as the right logistics and distribution channels to serve different ecosystem actors. It also has the right financial infrastructure to manage payments and financial benefits. Such big tech providers can deliver technology-agnostic services and augment those services with healthcare-specific capabilities to create a differentiated ecosystem. However, they depend on payers and healthcare providers to develop data curation strategies that can address issues of security, privacy and consent. Gaining the trust and confidence of the patients, who are not used to having big tech managing their points of care, would be key. This means that technology providers would have to partner with key payers and providers to build that trust before they can convince the rest of the ecosystem actors that they can orchestrate digitally enabled healthcare services across modalities of care.

The evolution toward ecosystem strategies presents an opportunity for providers and payers to increase their return on previous capital investments in digital technology, operational systems and human training and skill development. Large providers that also act as private payers and that own multiple primary care and hospital centers can act as ecosystem orchestrators for certain populations across the healthcare delivery cycle, but other medium and smaller providers will most probably participate in an ecosystem orchestrated by payers or digital technology providers. For providers that make a strategic choice to be a complementor in an ecosystem orchestrated by payers or even digital technology providers, it will be important to have a distinctive value proposition. Such a value proposition may include offering specialized services (e.g., robotic surgery) that others do not offer, something which would require combinations with other ecosystem actors toward new digital capabilities, as well as investments in new human skills. For example, Intuitive, the company that developed the Da Vinci robot, has engaged in extensive education programs and events for hospital executives, staff and surgeons.[89] These programs have a dual objective not only to train everyone that will be working with the Da Vinci robot, including ways of coordinating between them, but also to train the robot itself to improve its accuracy and effectiveness. Once again, there are complementarities in development that generate insights for other ecosystem actors to learn and produce yet new services and products.

New digital startups, medical device manufacturers and pharma and biotech organizations can act as complementors to different ecosystems because their capabilities are quite niche and specialized toward specific populations and types of care. However, these companies could play important complementor roles that could eventually grow into smaller ecosystems in and of themselves. For example, whole genome sequencing companies could evolve to create markets for genomic products and services. Illumina[90] is one such company that provides ecosystem-wide genomic data capabilities for healthcare providers, researchers and industry actors. Equally, data analytics and machine learning companies like Imagia[91] can play a critical role in converting underlying data to actionable insights for a variety of ecosystem actors. Pharma and biotech can also play a very important role in generating and storing medical data that could serve several different objectives, including diagnosis, but also medical research. As new technology capabilities mature, new digital startups, medical device manufacturers as well as pharma and biotech organizations can build on these capabilities to develop healthcare-specific insights. These insights can be provided to the patient in an efficient and actionable way, while also improving the quality of care.

Digital platform ecosystems hold opportunities to transform healthcare services, while improving health outcomes and delivering a personalized, integrated experience to patients. However, building successful ecosystems relies on aligning interests and coordinating with diverse stakeholders, while implementing several mechanisms to remove bottlenecks and leverage complementarities. This book will provide the tools with which to develop successful digital transformation strategies through an ecosystem approach.

Notes

1 Boh, W., Constantinides, P., Padmanabhan, B. and Viswanathan, S., 2023. Building digital resilience against major shocks. *MIS Quarterly*, 47(1), pp. 343–360.
2 Tangcharoensathien, V., Bassett, M.T., Meng, Q. and Mills, A., 2021. Are overwhelmed health systems an inevitable consequence of COVID-19? Experiences from China, Thailand, and New York State. *British Medical Journal*, 372, pp. 1-5; Trias-Llimós, S. and Bilal, U., 2020. Impact of the COVID-19 pandemic on life expectancy in Madrid (Spain). *Journal of Public Health*, 42(3), pp. 635–636; Vigo, D., Patten, S., Pajer, K., Krausz, M., Taylor, S., Rush, B., Raviola, G., Saxena, S., Thornicroft, G. and Yatham, L.N., 2020. Mental health of communities during the COVID-19 pandemic. *The Canadian Journal of Psychiatry*, 65(10), pp. 1–7.

3 See https://indianexpress.com/article/cities/mumbai/mumbai-faces-severe-shortage-of-ventilators-7288981/

4 Centers for Disease Control and Prevention on COVID-19 Racial and Ethnic Health Disparities https://www.cdc.gov/coronavirus/2019-ncov/community/health-equity/racial-ethnic-disparities/index.html

5 European Commission report "Health at a Glance: Europe 2020" https://ec.europa.eu/health/state/glance_en

6 WHO report on the COVID-19 global supply chain https://www.who.int/emergencies/diseases/novel-coronavirus-2019/COVID-19-operations

7 A commentary on the failed attempt of Sweden at achieving herd immunity https://www.reuters.com/article/uk-factcheck-prageru-sweden-herd-immunit-idUSKBN28C2R7; Modig, K., Ahlbom, A. and Ebeling, M., 2021. Excess mortality from COVID-19: weekly excess death rates by age and sex for Sweden and its most affected region. *European Journal of Public Health*, 31(1), pp. 17–22.

8 European Commission report "Health at a Glance: Europe 2020" https://ec.europa.eu/health/state/glance_en

9 American Hospital Association report here https://www.aha.org/issue-brief/2020-06-30-new-aha-report-finds-losses-deepen-hospitals-and-health-systems-due-COVID-19

10 Evergreen Life App. https://www.evergreen-life.co.uk/evergreen-life-app/

11 Amol Soin, M.D. and Laxmaiah Manchikanti, M.D., 2020. The effect of COVID-19 on interventional pain management practices: a physician burnout survey. *Pain Physician*, 23, pp. S271-S282; Nicola, M., Alsafi, Z., Sohrabi, C., Kerwan, A., Al-Jabir, A., Iosifidis, C., Agha, M. and Agha, R., 2020. The socio-economic implications of the coronavirus and COVID-19 pandemic: a review. *International Journal of Surgery*, 78, pp. 185-193.

12 Adesoye, T., Davis, C.H., Del Calvo, H., Shaikh, A.F., Chegireddy, V., Chan, E.Y., Martinez, S., Pei, K.Y., Zheng, F. and Tariq, N., 2021. Optimization of surgical resident safety and education during the COVID-19 pandemic – lessons learned. *Journal of Surgical Education*, 78(1), pp. 315–320.

13 Jackson, D., Bradbury-Jones, C., Baptiste, D., Gelling, L., Morin, K., Neville, S. and Smith, G.D., 2020. Life in the pandemic: some reflections on nursing in the context of COVID-19. *Journal of Clinical Nursing*, 29(13-14), pp. 2041-2043

14 WHO guidance on public health surveillance https://www.who.int/immunization/monitoring_surveillance/burden/vpd/en/

15 For example, see the Covid Symptom Tracker: https://covid.joinzoe.com/- developed by Kings College London; and the Private Kit Safe Paths: http://safepaths.mit.edu/ - developed by MIT; but also the collaboration between Apple and Google https://www.apple.com/newsroom/2020/04/apple-and-google-partner-on-COVID-19-contact-tracing-technology/

16 It should be noted here that South Korea was one of the few reported countries to have had data-sharing arrangements in place that made contact tracing possible and successful. https://www.newyorker.com/news/news-desk/seouls-radical-experiment-in-digital-contact-tracing

17 Rocklöv, J. and Sjödin, H., 2020. High population densities catalyse the spread of COVID-19. *Journal of travel medicine*, 27(3), pp. 1–2.

18 Shiau, S., Krause, K.D., Valera, P., Swaminathan, S. and Halkitis, P.N., 2020. The burden of COVID-19 in people living with HIV: a syndemic perspective. *AIDS and Behavior*, 24(8), pp. 2244–2249; Jay, J., Bor, J., Nsoesie, E.O., Lipson, S.K., Jones, D.K., Galea, S. and Raifman, J., 2020. Neighbourhood income and physical distancing during the COVID-19 pandemic in the United States. *Nature Human Behaviour*, 4(12), pp. 1294–1302; Ali, S., Asaria, M. and Stranges, S., 2020. COVID-19 and inequality: are we all in this together?. *Canadian Journal of Public Health*, 111(3), pp. 415–416.

19 Wymant, C., Ferretti, L., Tsallis, D., Charalambides, M., Abeler-Dörner, L., Bonsall, D., Hinch, R., Kendall, M., Milsom, L., Ayres, M. and Holmes, C., 2021. The epidemiological impact of the NHS COVID-19 App. *Nature* (2021). https://doi.org/10.1038/s41586-021-03606-z

20 Holtz, D., Zhao, M., Benzell, S.G., Cao, C.Y., Rahimian, M.A., Yang, J., Allen, J., Collis, A., Moehring, A., Sowrirajan, T. and Ghosh, D., 2020. Interdependence and the cost of uncoordinated responses to COVID-19. *Proceedings of the National Academy of Sciences*, 117(33), pp. 19837–19843.

21 Nsubuga, P., White, M.E., Thacker, S.B., Anderson, M.A., Blount, S.B., Broome, C.V., Chiller, T.M., Espitia, V., Imtiaz, R., Sosin, D. and Stroup, D.F., 2006. Public health surveillance: a tool for targeting and monitoring interventions, In Jamison, D.T., Breman, J.G., Measham, A.R., Alleyne, G., Claeson, M., Evans, D.B., Jha, P., Mills, A. and Musgrove, P. (eds.), *Disease Control Priorities in Developing Countries*, pp. 997–1018. 2nd edition, The International Bank for Reconstruction and Development/The World Bank Group. https://pubmed.ncbi.nlm.nih.gov/21250345/

22 Phalkey, R.K., Yamamoto, S., Awate, P. and Marx, M., 2015. Challenges with the implementation of an Integrated Disease Surveillance and Response (IDSR) system: systematic review of the lessons learned. *Health Policy and Planning*, 30(1), pp.131–143.

23 Bashshur, R. and Shannon, G.W., 2009. *History of Telemedicine: Evolution, Context, and Transformation* (Vol. 2009). New Rochelle, NY: Mary Ann Liebert.

24 See https://www.appannie.com/en/insights/market-data/at-home-fitness-apps-in-demand-coronavirus/

25 See https://www.appannie.com/en/insights/mobile-minute/telehealth-apps-grow-amid-social-distancing/

26 Black Book Market Research report on COVID-19 https://blackbookmarketresearch.com/administrator/img/0188_SGP_COVID-19%20Market%20Pulse_r2.pdf

27 Fierce Health report on telehealth https://www.fiercehealthcare.com/practices/half-physicians-now-using-telehealth-as-covid-changes-practice-operations

28 See https://ir.teladochealth.com/news-and-events/investor-news/press-release-details/2023/Teladoc-Health-Reports-Fourth-Quarter-and-Full-Year-2022-Results/default.aspx

29 See https://doctorcareanywhere.com/media/4622/fy22-preliminary-final-report.pdf

30 See https://www.ft.com/partnercontent/ping-an-insurance/building-healthcares-future.html

31 Topol, E., 2012. *The Creative Destruction of Medicine: How the Digital Revolution Will Create Better Health Care*. Basic Books, New York, USA

32 Kwon, S.Y., 2016. Regulating personalized medicine. *Berkeley Technology Law Journal*, 31(2), pp. 931–960; Wadmann, S. and Hauge, A.M., 2021. Strategies of stratification: regulating market access in the era of personalized medicine. *Social Studies of Science*, 51(4), pp. 628-653

33 Attia, P. 2023. *Outlive: The Science and Art of Longevity*. Ebury Publishing, London UK

34 I thank Professor Elena Karahanna of the University of Georgia for this point.

35 Matchar, D.B., McCrory, D.C., Orlando, L.A., Patel, M.R., Patel, U.D., Patwardhan, M.B., Powers, B., Samsa, G.P. and Gray, R.N., 2008. Systematic review: comparative effectiveness of angiotensin-converting enzyme inhibitors and angiotensin II receptor blockers for treating essential hypertension. *Annals of Internal Medicine*, 148(1), pp. 16–29; Hernandez, A.F., Hammill, B.G., O'connor, C.M., Schulman, K.A., Curtis, L.H. and Fonarow, G.C., 2009. Clinical effectiveness of beta-blockers in heart failure: findings from the OPTIMIZE-HF (Organized Program to Initiate Lifesaving Treatment in Hospitalized Patients with Heart Failure) Registry. *Journal of the American College of Cardiology*, 53(2), pp. 184–192.

36 Pirmohamed, M., James, S., Meakin, S., Green, C., Scott, A.K., Walley, T.J., Farrar, K., Park, B.K. and Breckenridge, A.M., 2004. Adverse drug reactions as cause of admission to hospital: prospective analysis of 18 820 patients. *BMJ*, 329(7456), pp. 15–19; Davies, E.C., Green, C.F., Taylor, S., Williamson, P.R., Mottram, D.R. and Pirmohamed, M., 2009. Adverse drug reactions in hospital in-patients: a prospective analysis of 3695 patient-episodes. *PLoS One*, 4(2), p. e4439.

37 Chyka, P.A., 2000. How many deaths occur annually from adverse drug reactions in the United States?. *The American Journal of Medicine*, 109(2), pp. 122–130.

38 Attia, P., 2023. *Outlive: The Science and Art of Longevity*. p. 31.Ebury Publishing, London UK

39 Cirulli, E.T. and Goldstein, D.B., 2010. Uncovering the roles of rare variants in common disease through whole-genome sequencing. *Nature Reviews Genetics*, 11(6), pp. 415–425; Kuroda, M., Ohta, T., Uchiyama, I., Baba, T., Yuzawa, H., Kobayashi, I., Cui, L., Oguchi, A., Aoki, K.I., Nagai, Y. and Lian, J., 2001. Whole genome sequencing of meticillin-resistant Staphylococcus aureus. *The Lancet*, 357(9264), pp. 1225–1240; Roach, J.C., Glusman, G., Smit, A.F., Huff, C.D., Hubley, R., Shannon, P.T., Rowen, L., Pant, K.P., Goodman, N., Bamshad, M. and Shendure, J., 2010. Analysis of genetic inheritance in a family quartet by whole-genome sequencing. *Science*, 328(5978), pp. 636–639.

40 See the Human Genome factsheet https://www.genome.gov/about-genomics/fact-sheets/Sequencing-Human-Genome-cost

41 Dante Labs currently offers whole human genome sequencing starting from $599 https://www.dantelabs.com/

42 Illumina https://www.illumina.com/

43 Jain, M., Koren, S., Miga, K.H., Quick, J., Rand, A.C., Sasani, T.A., Tyson, J.R., Beggs, A.D., Dilthey, A.T., Fiddes, I.T. and Malla, S., 2018. Nanopore sequencing and assembly of a human genome with ultra-long reads. *Nature biotechnology*, 36(4), pp. 338–345; see also https://www.labiotech.eu/more-news/oxford-nanopore-whole-genome-sequencing/

44 https://www.genomicsengland.co.uk/about-genomics-england/the-100000-genomes-project/

45 Genomics England https://www.genomicsengland.co.uk/understanding-genomics/

46 Attia, P. 2023. *Outlive: The Science and Art of Longevity. Ebury Publishing, London UK*

47 Hou, Y.C.C., Yu, H.C., Martin, R., Schenker-Ahmed, N.M., Hicks, M., Cirulli, E.T., Cohen, I.V., Jonsson, T.J., Heister, R., Napier, L. and Swisher, C.L., 2018. Precision medicine advancements using whole genome sequencing, noninvasive whole body imaging, and functional diagnostics. *bioRxiv*, p. 497560; also see https://humanlongevity.com/ (previously called HealthNucleus). https://www.biorxiv.org/content/10.1101/497560v1.full.pdf

48 See for example https://www.diabeteseducator.org/danatech/glucose-monitoring/continuous-glucose-monitors-(cgm) for a list of continuous glucose monitors.

49 https://quantifiedself.com/about/what-is-quantified-self/

50 Holmström, I. and Röing, M., 2010. The relation between patient-centeredness and patient empowerment: a discussion on concepts. *Patient Education and Counseling*, 79(2), pp. 167–172.

51 Feng, S., Mäntymäki, M., Dhir, A. and Salmela, H., 2021. How self-tracking and the quantified self promote health and well-being: systematic review. *Journal of Medical Internet Research*, 23(9), p. e25171.

52 Sharon, T., 2017. Self-tracking for health and the quantified self: re-articulating autonomy, solidarity, and authenticity in an age of personalized healthcare. *Philosophy & Technology*, 30(1), pp. 93–121.

53 https://blueprint.bryanjohnson.co/

54 https://www.bloomberg.com/news/features/2023-01-25/anti-aging-techniques-taken-to-extreme-by-bryan-johnson

55 Lupton, D., 2013. The digitally engaged patient: self-monitoring and self-care in the digital health era. *Social Theory & Health*, 11(3), pp. 256–270. p. 256.

56 van Uden-Kraan, C.F., Drossaert, C.H., Taal, E., Shaw, B.R., Seydel, E.R. and van de Laar, M.A., 2008. Empowering processes and outcomes of participation in online support groups for patients with breast cancer, arthritis, or fibromyalgia. *Qualitative Health Research*, 18(3), pp. 405–417.

57 Boh, W., Constantinides, P., Padmanabhan, B. and Viswanathan, S., 2023. Building digital resilience against major shocks. *MIS Quarterly*, 47(1), pp. 343–360.

58 Christensen, C., 1997. *The Innovator's Dilemma*. Harvard Business School Press. Boston USA

59 Parker G.G., Van Alstyne M.W., Choudary S.P., 2016. *Platform Revolution: How Networked Markets Are Transforming the Economy and How to Make Them Work for You*. New York: W. W. Norton; Constantinides, P., Henfridsson, O. and Parker, G.G., 2018. Platforms and infrastructures in the digital age. *Information Systems Research*, 29(2), pp. 381–400.

60 Jacobides, M.G., Cennamo, C. and Gawer, A., 2018. Towards a theory of ecosystems. *Strategic Management Journal*, 39(8), pp. 2255–2276; Adner, R., 2017. Ecosystem as structure: an actionable construct for strategy. *Journal of Management*, 43(1), pp. 39–58.

61 https://www.instadeep.com/2020/11/biontech-and-instadeep-announce-strategic-collaboration-and-form-ai-innovation-lab-to-develop-novel-immunotherapies/

62 https://hbr.org/2022/04/will-mrna-technology-companies-spawn-innovation-ecosystems

63 Teece, D.J. 2009. *Dynamic Capabilities and Strategic Management: Organizing for Innovation and Growth*. Oxford University Press. Oxford UK

64 Arthur, W.B., 2009. *The Nature of Technology: What It Is and How It Evolves*. Penguin Books; Baldwin, C.Y. and Clark, K.B., 2000. *Design Rules – The Power of Modularity*, Cambridge, MA: MIT Press.

65 Baldwin, C.Y. and Clark, K.B., 2000. *Design Rules – The Power of Modularity*, Cambridge, MA: MIT Press; Hanseth, O. and Lyytinen, K., 2010. Design theory for dynamic complexity in

information infrastructures: the case of building Internet. *Journal of Information Technology* 25(1) 1–19; Schilling, M.A., 2000. Towards a general modular systems theory and its application to interfirm product modularity, *Academy of Management Review* 25(2), pp. 312–334; Simon, H.A., 1996. *The Sciences of the Artificial*. 3rd edition. MIT Press. Boston USA

66 Yoo, Y., Henfridsson, O. and Lyytinen, K., 2010. The new organizing logic of digital innovation: an agenda for information systems research. *Information Systems Research*, 21(4), pp. 724–735.

67 Baldwin, C.Y., Clark, K.B. and Clark, K.B., 2000. *Design Rules: The Power of Modularity* (Vol. 1). MIT Press., Boston USA

68 Arthur, W.B., 2009. *The Nature of Technology: What It Is and How It Evolves*. Simon & Schuster., London UK

69 I thank Professor Arun Rai of Georgia State University for this point.

70 Williams, I., Allen, K. and Plahe, G., 2019. Reports of rationing from the neglected realm of capital investment: responses to resource constraint in the English National Health Service. *Social Science & Medicine*, 225, pp. 1–8.

71 https://www.forbes.com/sites/sachinjain/2023/04/24/can-we-avoid-the-impending-healthcare-workforce-labor-shortage/?sh=671411c9fdb5; https://www.mckinsey.com/industries/healthcare/our-insights/the-gathering-storm-the-uncertain-future-of-us-healthcare

72 Kretschmer, T., Leiponen, A., Schilling, M. and Vasudeva, G., 2022. Platform ecosystems as meta-organizations: implications for platform strategies. *Strategic Management Journal*, 43(3), pp. 405–424; Adner, R., 2017. Ecosystem as structure: an actionable construct for strategy. *Journal of Management*, 43(1), pp. 39–58; Jacobides, M.G., Cennamo, C. and Gawer, A., 2018. Towards a theory of ecosystems. *Strategic Management Journal*, 39(8), pp. 2255–2276.

73 https://www.doccla.com/

74 Constantinides, P., Henfridsson, O. and Parker, G.G., 2018. Platforms and infrastructures in the digital age. *Information Systems Research*, 29(2), pp. 381–400.

75 https://aws.amazon.com/about-aws/whats-new/2012/04/19/introducing-aws-marketplace/

76 https://aws.amazon.com/health/

77 Lusch, R.F. and Nambisan, S., 2015. Service innovation: a service-dominant logic perspective. *MIS Quarterly*, 39(1), pp. 155–175; Bowman, C. and Ambrosini, V., 2000. Value creation versus value capture: towards a coherent definition of value in strategy. *British Journal of Management*, 11(1), pp. 1–15.

78 Lusch, R.F. and Nambisan, S., 2015. Service innovation: a service-dominant logic perspective. *MIS Quarterly*, 39(1), pp. 155–175; Bowman, C. and Ambrosini, V., 2000. Value creation versus value capture: towards a coherent definition of value in strategy. *British Journal of Management*, 11(1), pp. 1–15.

79 https://www.babylonhealth.com/us/what-we-offer/chatbot

80 https://covid.randox.com/day-2-test-at-home/

81 https://covid.randox.com/certifly-app-download/

82 https://www.england.nhs.uk/contact-us/privacy-notice/how-we-use-your-information/our-services/primary-care-commissioning/

83 Dr OnDemand, Virtual Care Utilization report https://info.doctorondemand.com/virtual_care_utilization_report

84 Credit Suisse. 2019. Healthcare transformation. https://www.credit-suisse.com/media/assets/corporate/docs/about-us/research/publications/csri-healthcare-information.pdf

85 https://www.alibabacloud.com/solutions/intelligence-brain/medical#f9

86 Credit Suisse. 2019. Healthcare transformation. https://www.credit-suisse.com/media/assets/corporate/docs/about-us/research/publications/csri-healthcare-information.pdf

87 Examples include Apple Health, Samsung Health and Google Fit.

88 Some examples include Iora Health https://www.iorahealth.com and Omada Health https://www.omadahealth.com/

89 https://www.intuitive.com/en-us/healthcare-professionals/hospitals

90 https://www.illumina.com/

91 https://imagia.com/

2 Complexity in Healthcare Services

Chapter 1 has pointed at the multiple ecosystems, both small and large, currently emerging around healthcare services. Many of these ecosystems are products of digital disruption and transformation as in the case of ecosystems orchestrated by Teladoc and Ping An Good Doctor, while others are products of longer systemic transformation through patient empowerment and personalized medicine driven by the proliferation of personal smart devices. However, not all patients have access to these ecosystems, and many experience an increasing complexity in healthcare services including rising and variable costs for treatment options, diagnostics and hospital care. There is also a rising doctor and carer burnout in national health systems due to increased workloads, low numbers of staff and other resource constraints, which contribute to medical errors and poor performance, feeding into a vicious cycle of increased costs. These complex challenges are pounded by the lack of interoperability between information systems and applications, as well as issues of data access. Finally, there are ethical and regulatory challenges to governing data generated through, and accessed by, new innovations in healthcare. Different types of organizations from healthcare service providers to device manufacturers, small biotech companies and insurance companies need to address these complex challenges by engaging in large-scale transformation programs. This chapter provides an in-depth discussion of these challenges to set the ground for understanding organizational change and digital transformation.

2.1 Health Spending, Technology Diffusion and the Costs and Outcomes of Healthcare Services

Healthcare spending has increased around the world, and although some benefits have been gained, there have been substantial concerns among private and public payers, as well as other healthcare organizations, as to whether financing this continuous increase is sustainable. The rising cost of healthcare has been a major concern in most countries, since addressing health spending growth without cutting other public programs would require a significant increase in taxes.[1] Moreover, a recent World Health Organization report[2] shows that, in most countries, more than 30 percent of healthcare spending is wasted on services with unclear benefits on outcomes. Thus, even if countries continue to find ways to keep financing this growth, the long-term benefits are unclear.

Historical evidence shows that a primary determinant of health spending growth is the development and diffusion of new medical knowledge, applications and technologies to address a healthcare problem. Take the example of the recent COVID-19 pandemic. The Sars-Cov-2 virus emerged as a new healthcare problem that required

DOI: 10.4324/9781032619569-3

the medical knowledge of previous coronaviruses, the application of genetic testing and analysis and the development of new biotechnology such as mRNA vaccines. New knowledge and technology may lead to new innovations in existing healthcare services influencing demand for new complementary services. The accelerated use and success of mRNA technology during the COVID-19 pandemic is currently pushing forward further applications not just to vaccination, but also protein-replacement therapy, gene editing and cellular reprogramming and engineering for chronic and rare diseases.[3]

Such innovations in medical technology increase demand for new applications and impact healthcare spending. For example, innovations in laparoscopic cholecystectomy in the early 1990s led to a 60 percent increase in its use.[4] Prior to the innovation, many asymptomatic or mildly symptomatic individuals may not have been treated because the risk and morbidity associated with previous treatment options exceeded that associated with the disease. Because of the growing number of cholecystectomies, but also because of increased diagnostic testing associated with the procedure, health spending also grew. Interestingly, more recent studies have also found that laparoscopic cholecystectomy is associated with adverse effects including biliary and vascular injury,[5] which leads to additional treatment and thus further increasing costs. Certainly, the new innovations substitute existing knowledge, applications and technologies that offset some of the additional costs incurred. Despite complementing and substituting existing services, however, what matters the most for overall spending growth is how the new innovations change use patterns with respect to the relative costs of the services. This is where complexity rises.

The cost for new services will vary depending on the price parameters set by different payers and their insurance plans. For example, some insurance plans set price rationing mechanisms such as a coinsurance rate (a portion of the medical cost a patient pays after the deductible has been met), while others set condition-specific limits on the amount of care patients can consume. Both approaches are dynamically adapted based on demand and supply shocks to healthcare services (e.g., fewer patients choosing a particular service; fewer providers offering that service). In other words, even though there may be new innovations that may impact spending growth, as discussed above, healthcare spending may also be determined by managerial fiat. In fact, there is a dynamic relationship between incentives for technology development subsidized by certain price rationing mechanisms and (dis-)incentives on the amount of care patients consume as conditioned by limits set by their insurance plans. For example, the use of coinsurance for expensive drugs rather than the use of co-payments for most other drugs impacts the incentives to develop such drugs.[6] Other adverse effects include cases where some technologies benefit a subset of the population disproportionately, but with health insurance plans increasing demand to a larger population and potentially causing an overall decrease in welfare.[7] Indeed, the widespread use of health insurance with specific price rationing mechanisms can lead not only to lower welfare but also to moral hazard and adverse selection of new innovations, whether those are new diagnostic and treatment procedures including new drugs or other types of healthcare services. The degree of such adverse effects varies across regions due to supply and demand factors, where economic stability (e.g., employment, income) impacts access to healthcare services, but also provision of those.[8] However, managerial fiat based on supply-driven forms of organizing healthcare services impacts how demand-driven innovation is diffused across different segments of the population.

One of the key efforts of health systems is to optimize the utilization of healthcare services, as a way of achieving equity, while also ensuring that there is efficient use of scarce resources. This effort is filled with trade-offs, however, because no two individuals have the same needs and no matter how well economic models are designed, some individuals will always end up paying for services they never consume or do not need because of the process by which these offerings are made available to them. Some technology and medical applications will end up being more aggressively promoted than others based on aggregated benefits for the population. For example, the National Institute for Health and Clinical Excellence (NICE) that offers guidance on the use of new and existing medicines and treatments within the National Health Service (NHS) in England and Wales is much less likely to recommend that an intervention should receive government reimbursement if the cost per quality-adjusted life years (QALY) of that intervention is high as compared to if it is low. According to NICE, "one quality-adjusted life year (QALY) is equal to 1 year of life in perfect health. QALYs are calculated by estimating the years of life remaining for a patient following a particular treatment or intervention and weighting each year with a quality-of-life score (on a 0 to 1 scale)".[9] Interventions costing the NHS less than £30,000 per QALY gained are deemed cost-effective and can be recommended for funding, while those that cost more than this are not. QALYs are calculated through contingent evaluation methods that involve surveys of people asking them to choose between, for example, the certainty of remaining in a particular health state versus taking a gamble of either being in full health or risking death (what is called the "standard gamble") or between living in an impaired health state for the rest of their life (e.g., type 2 diabetes) versus living in full health for a shorter period of time (what is called the "time trade-off").[10] While there are obvious benefits to eliciting valuations of health states through QALYs from patients and the public as opposed to more expert parties, evidence shows that such valuations overestimate losses and underestimate adaptations to health states.[11] Such valuations are based on the premise of predicting a desired outcome, as opposed to understanding the actual experience of patients with a health state.

Evidently, developing health policies to account for new innovations in medical knowledge and technology, determining the appropriate price rationing mechanisms for insurance plans and calculating QALYs based on the perceived and expected health states of the population are no easy tasks. Institutes such as NICE acting on behalf of a national payer or commercial payers acting on behalf of their shareholders are constantly trying to optimize their economic models to manage the trade-offs between cost-efficiency and equity, but the reality is that these models will often only serve specific segments of the population, while producing poor or no value for other segments. These dynamics usually end up with higher costs for the patients themselves, while leaving room for counterproductive behaviors, including contracts between insurance companies and hospitals on markup prices for services[12] that only encourage "overtesting, over-diagnosing and overtreatment".[13] A recent report by the *New York Times* in collaboration with the University of Maryland in Baltimore took advantage of a recent federal regulation that orders hospitals to publish a complete list of the prices they negotiate with private insurers. The report found great price variation even within the same hospital.[14] For example, the report showed that an MRI at Boston, Massachusetts-based Mass General was $1,019 for patients covered by a Cigna plan. But that price shot up to $3,101 for patients covered by an Aetna plan and $3,809 for those covered by a Humana plan. The American Hospital Association has been very critical of this new regulation with some hospital associations jointly suing the federal government and the Centers for Medicare & Medicaid Services (CMS) that proposed it, to block it. Despite losing to the lawsuit and the appeals, some hospitals have simply decided to ignore the requirement and post nothing.[15] This is not just a US problem. A European study of the costs and survival of hospital-admitted stroke patients varied across Europe because of differences in unit costs and resource use.[16] Similar findings were reported in a Chinese study.[17] Thus, once again, supply-driven forms of organizing healthcare services affect how patients access services and what they pay for those, often with very little choice.

In recent years, there have been several initiatives from professional associations and patient advocate groups such as Choosing Wisely[18] to identify which medical procedures and technology applications provide minimal or no benefit and at what cost. The Choosing Wisely website provides lists of recommended treatments by medical condition for both patients and clinicians and has already informed several studies. One such study[19] used Medicare data from 2006 to 2011 to create claims-based algorithms to measure the prevalence of 11 low-value services identified by Choosing Wisely and to examine geographic variation across hospital referral regions (HRRs). The study found that "the national average annual prevalence of the selected Choosing Wisely low-value services ranged from 1.2% (e.g., upper urinary tract imaging in men with benign prostatic hyperplasia) to 46.5% (e.g., preoperative cardiac testing for low-risk, non-cardiac procedures)". The study also found that "regional characteristics associated with higher use of low-value services included greater overall per capita spending, a higher specialist to primary care ratio and higher proportion of minority beneficiaries".[20] Arguably such initiatives as Choosing Wisely are important for changing health *policies*. However, changing health *practices* is no easy task, particularly when a low-value service may be highly profitable for healthcare professionals or for the organization that employs them.[21] Payment reforms such as pay-for-performance have been introduced to change the practices of healthcare professionals and organizations; however, there is no standard system that determines what a hospital charges for a particular service or procedure. Many factors figure into hospital pricing, including an individual's health circumstances, "best practices" adopted by health providers, operating room and post-surgical costs, medications and doctors' and specialists' fees. For example, if one patient's recovery from an operation takes place in an Intensive Care Unit (ICU) and another patient's recovery takes place in a recovery room, costs can vary by thousands of dollars, even if the two patients' surgeries were similar. So regardless of a hospital's published fee schedules for a service or procedure, there is no reliable way to assess a patient's final hospital costs.[22]

Variation in costs is only one dimension of the problem. Another is unclear benefits based on limited evidence for services provided. For example, both female and male cancer screening conducted through mammography scans and prostate biopsies, respectively, have very high costs and very little outcome improvement. On the one hand, data on women who have mammography each year since 1975 show that "they are more likely to have breast cancer that was over diagnosed than to have earlier detection of a tumor that was destined to become large".[23] The false positives often lead to additional tests such as biopsies and unnecessary surgeries or radiation therapy. On the other hand, "the usefulness and desirability of routine PSA-based screening" for prostate cancer in men are still unclear after 25 years and large trials, and evidence suggests that "its net benefit is unlikely to be more than marginal, whereas the harms are proven and substantial".[24] In medicine, professional guidelines are particularly important because they define the standard of care and ways for assessing cases of malpractice.[25] Guidelines are another dimension of population-level decisions that dictate when tests such as pelvic exams, annual physicals, PSA tests and PAP smears should be done, as well as how certain medical conditions should be diagnosed and classified, even though, often there would be limited data to do so.

Evidently, the constantly rising cost for healthcare services, the use of resources to perform various procedures and the unclear outcomes are the consequence of decisions based on population averages and broad guidelines that do not consider the specific case of individual patients. Lack of patient choice but, most importantly, lack of intelligence in decisions across different levels from policy organizations and payers to health providers and individual healthcare professionals lead to unnecessary interventions and waste of resources. These challenges are primarily observed in supply-driven forms of organizing healthcare services that only add to the vicious cycle of clinical inefficacy and moral hazard for the patients, but also the burnout of healthcare professionals, which increases medical errors and impacts performance.

2.2   Burnout, Medical Errors and Poor Performance

Burnout is a work-related hazard that is prevalent among those working in people-oriented professions such as healthcare. Burnout is defined as "a psychological syndrome emerging as a prolonged response to chronic interpersonal stressors on the job".[26] There are three dimensions of burnout, including an "overwhelming exhaustion, feelings of cynicism and detachment from the job, and a sense of ineffectiveness and lack of accomplishment".[26]

The rate of burnout among healthcare professionals tends to be reported in the moderate to high levels, and it is generally believed that the burnout risk in healthcare is higher than in the general working population.[27] The 2020 Medscape National Physician Burnout and Suicide Report found evidence of burnout across 29 medical specialities, from urology, neurology, general surgery and psychiatry.[28] Other studies from Europe have pointed at significantly higher levels of burnout for critical care workers working at intensive care units and emergency dispatch.[29] Yet, other studies point at differences in burnout according to the career stage of healthcare professionals.[30] Estimates also vary depending on which dimension of burnout is being considered (i.e., exhaustion, detachment or professional inefficacy) and what degree of burnout is considered important. For example, the European General Practice Research Network Burnout Study Group found that while 12 percent of participants suffered from burnout in all three dimensions, 43 percent scored high for emotional exhaustion, 35 percent for detachment and 32 percent for professional inefficacy.[31] In the UK, burnout is common among healthcare professionals, with prevalence estimates predominantly ranging between 40 and 60 percent across the three dimensions,[32] which are comparable to studies of burnout in the Middle East.[33] Overall, evidence suggests that many healthcare professionals will experience burnout in their careers and that burnout can have devastating consequences for affected professionals, their colleagues and their patients.

There are various sources of burnout reported in the aforementioned studies, from individual aspirations not met, to the blame culture within the professional setting, to the burden of new technologies and changes in work environments, as well as poor leadership. These sources are deeply embedded in the training and education, as well as the working environment of healthcare professionals and are often reinforced throughout their careers. For example, poor learning environments where there is inadequate supervision[34] as well as disorganized hospital settings with bottlenecks in the patient journey are associated with burnout and medical errors.[35] The problem of medical errors is highly interdependent with the discussion in the previous section on the rising costs of healthcare services, the waste of resources and the unclear outcomes for patients.

Medical errors range from medication errors, patient misidentification and errors or delays in diagnosis.[36] In addition to these errors that may be made by many different healthcare professionals, errors made by surgeons include wrong site or wrong procedure surgeries,[37] or errors in judgment that lead to either an unnecessary operation or delay of a necessary operation.[38] Such errors can be substantial and lead to dramatic consequences for the patient, but also the healthcare provider.[39] Studies show that errors can increase the prevalence of burnout on healthcare professionals that can last for years after the error occurred, feeding into a vicious cycle of further errors and burnout.[40]

Research has proposed several interventions for preventing and reducing burnout and medical error from structural interventions within the work environment, consisting of shortened rotation length,[41] various modifications to clinical work processes[42] and shortened resident shifts.[43] Other studies involved individual-focused interventions, consisting of facilitated small group curricula,[44] stress management and self-care training[45] and communication skills training by means of reporting burnout and avoiding errors.[46] Although many of these interventions focus on building individual-level resilience[47] as a preventative strategy against burnout, more recent research has also stressed the importance of system-level interventions to neutralize or reduce the impact of medical errors made by individuals.[48] Some sources of burnout and medical error should be addressed at the hospital level, professional body (e.g., Association of Surgeons) or even national level, where broader policies can be introduced.

For example, financial incentives based on performance have been proposed as a method for improving the quality of care and reducing medical errors by national payers, HMO and commercial payers.[49] However, as discussed in the previous section, such performance-based incentives can generate adverse effects. Indeed, research into the dynamic relationship between intrinsic motivation (e.g., enjoying one's job by performing creative tasks) and extrinsic incentives (e.g., financial incentives) found that the former matters more for higher quality performance, whereas the latter matters more for higher quantity performance.[50] This finding is in line with the discussion in the previous section and points to the fact that motivation should be considered by means of what it is supposed to address. This research has found that intrinsic motivation – the type of motivation that could prevent and reduce burnout and medical errors – is little impacted by extrinsic incentives. "However, incentive contingency has a very strong link to intrinsic motivation (r = .78): More controlling (directly salient) incentives are associated with lower intrinsic motivation, while less controlling (indirectly salient) incentives have a positive link".[50] In other words, when extrinsic incentives are present but only indirectly salient to performance, intrinsic motivation can have a higher impact on performance. Thus, designing policies for improving the quality of the performance should focus on the process of care not the outcome. This would help reduce medical errors while amplifying the intrinsic motivation and thus preventing and reducing burnout. It would also help avoiding counterproductive behaviors that are usually associated with performance-contingent incentives.[51]

As studies have shown, increasing the quality of performance while reducing burnout and errors does not depend just on measurement, practices and rules, nor does it depend on any specific improvement methods. It depends on achieving a safety culture.[52] Safety culture is one aspect of an organization's culture and refers to the shared values, beliefs, norms and procedures related to enacting an organization's safety among members of an organization, unit or team, including, in the context of healthcare, the safety of patients. Within healthcare organizations, safety culture influences the behaviors of healthcare professionals and other staff by providing cues about the relative priority of safety compared with other goals such as productivity and efficiency. Studies show that safety culture is related to such behaviors as error reporting, reductions in adverse events and reduced mortality, thus helping to reduce burnout and medical error while promoting the quality of performance.[53]

Achieving a safety culture, however, requires major transformation. Too many healthcare organizations suffer from hierarchical structures that are deficient in developing mutual respect, teamwork and transparency. Mechanisms for ensuring accountability are weak and ambiguous, and few organizations have the capacity to learn and change. Most do not recognize that safety should be a precondition, not a priority or that fulfilling the interests of their patients in safe care and of their staff in a safe workplace will enhance productivity and profitability. Many healthcare professionals do not know how to be team players and regard others as assistants. Finally, patients are seldom included in organizational planning or in the analysis of adverse events that have harmed them.[54]

All these situational aspects of safety culture can be unearthed and analyzed through a collection of data on an organization's policies, operating procedures and workflow systems, but also performance data within and across functional units, as well as data on patient outcomes. Such data analysis would help to examine the reciprocal relationship between the organization's safety management systems and the way those systems are perceived and experienced by individuals, EHRgroups and functional units. "It appears useful to examine the degree to which safety management systems actually influence people's behaviour, and vice-versa, at the strategic, tactical and operational levels of organisations".[55] This brings us to the next challenge, namely, the challenge of interoperability between information systems and applications, as well as the issues this generates for data access.

2.3 The Challenge of Interoperability and Data Access

Some estimates show that there are about 2,314 exabytes of data generated globally each year.[56] These data include patient clinical data (i.e., electronic health records (EHRs) including imaging and other device data), demographic and logistic data (e.g., scheduling), financial claims and payments, inventory and ordering, registry and other types of operational data, performance data on organizational, group and individual practices, macro- and micro-economic data including social determinants from population health and from national and private payers. Increasingly, these data also include omics data[57] from heterogeneous sources such as partner organizations (e.g., genomic, pharma and biotech organizations) and even data generated from patients through their personal devices. Even though, today, EHRs are increasingly paperless and a level of integration across different types of systems has been achieved by migrating to cloud models and application programming interfaces (API), there are still significant challenges to achieving seamless access to different types of data. These challenges include a lack of agreement about existing standards that would help achieve interoperability across healthcare information systems and applications, as well as issues of data quality.

Since the late 1990s, there have been numerous national and regional initiatives to develop a set of standards that would help integrate fragmented information systems into a common information infrastructure.[58] To achieve this, standards and systems need to be interoperable. Interoperability is used to "describe systems and services that are connected and can work together seamlessly and effectively, while maintaining patient and professional confidentiality, privacy and security".[59] At the technical level, interoperability enables one system or application to securely communicate data to and receive data from another, while using standardized definitions from publicly available value sets and coding vocabularies. Interoperability also includes governance, policy, social, legal and organizational considerations to facilitate the secure, seamless and timely communication and use of data both within and between organizations, entities and individuals. These considerations enable trust and integration between end-user processes and workflows.[60] There are, however, several barriers to achieving interoperability.

To achieve interoperability across information systems, coordinated action is required between actors. Such coordinated action often takes place through either a top-down or a bottom-up approach.

On the one hand, countries with a strong reliance on public health services like the English NHS have complex national governance structures that inevitably encourage a top-down system architecture, standards compliance and procurement process. The central vision of the English NHS' National Program for IT (NPfIT) was to standardize the previously fragmented IT delivery in all NHS organizations by introducing an integrated infrastructure.[61] This ambitious and wide-ranging information strategy included a vision of lifelong EHRs for every person in the country, and 24/7 online access to patient records and information about best clinical practice, for all NHS clinicians, enabling "genuinely seamless care for patients through GPs, hospitals and community services".[62] From the very start, the NPfIT was met with plenty of clinical unrest, delays, cost overruns and paring back of promised functionality, culminating in political demands to shut down the program.[63] Independent reviews of the NPfIT found that the main reason for this failure was that the complexity of the English NHS made it impossible to just impose a unified, national IT system from the top.[64] In a top-down approach, existing systems that do not comply with national standards are typically shut down and replaced by compliant ones. However, the new compliant systems may not fit local needs as well as the systems they replace. There is also the additional cost of staff retraining and workflow adjustment, with the risk of introducing unexpected errors into the care process. A top-down, centralized approach has limited capacity to adapt quickly to emerging health service delivery challenges and, thus, becomes increasingly out of step with service needs. Workarounds to make the aging systems meet emerging needs will start adding up but will inevitably become unmanageable local variations to what was intended to be a singular national system.[65]

On the other hand, countries with a healthy mix of private and public health services like the USA have embarked on a totally different, bottom-up approach to designing health information infrastructures. Service providers have formed regional coalitions to interconnect their existing systems as best they can into health information exchanges (HIEs). The expectation is that regional HIEs will eventually aggregate into a national system.[66] A bottom-up decentralized approach to developing health information systems has been adopted in many parts of the world.[67] However, although maintaining many disassociated information systems provides flexibility to meet a diverse variety of local healthcare needs, this flexibility also has some drawbacks.

To start with, most of these health information systems are designed and structured to meet the unique needs of each healthcare organization. Planning for interoperability with external systems is generally a low priority in the development process. As a result, health data is often collected in an inconsistent manner from one organization to another. Incompatible data models may make reconciling the same information across different systems arbitrarily complex. In turn, by preserving local systems, weaker national systems are produced that generate more interoperability issues and data quality problems. The presence of interoperability standards can minimize some of these risks, but at its extreme, a bottom-up strategy sees standards development and compliance as largely a voluntary affair. This means that governments become disinterested in bottom-up strategies since they are unlikely to be closely aligned with national policy goals. This often prevents the information systems of separate organizations from corresponding with each other successfully. The lack of standardization that results from this approach makes it difficult to assemble the data from these fragmented local databases.

These interoperability challenges create inefficiencies for healthcare providers, as well as the relationships between payers and patients and all the challenges discussed in the previous section regarding burnout, medical errors and poor performance outcomes. The infrastructure of many healthcare organizations is not directly interacting with patients and other healthcare organizations, which means that there are a lot of supporting technologies that are added onto this infrastructure by means of filling the gaps. Certainly, there are a lot of different technology providers currently trying to address the interoperability challenge but with varied approaches. These approaches vary from HIE, healthcare integration engines and EHR marketplaces.

First, HIEs facilitate data exchange in a "middle-out" approach[68] within a network of organizations, communities, states or regions.[69] HIEs may include healthcare providers, payers and other healthcare organizations to establish the governance and technical aspects of data exchange. As such, HIEs standardize data across organizations. HIEs were born out of regional health information organizations that helped connected providers that used different EHR systems to interact through a central information exchange. By using common standards provided by standards development organizations such as HL7 (Health Level 7), SNOMED (Systematized Nomenclature of Medicine), and CDISC (Clinical Data Interchange Standards Consortium), these HIEs help provide standardized data across the organizations that participate in the HIEs. However, what these HIEs do not provide is a scalable managed service that can add or remove connections to new actors on-demand. Each time a new participant joins the network, the HIE need to manually integrate their data and (possibly conflicting) standards to the rest of the participants. It is, thus, a highly centralized approach that lacks agility and flexibility. A new actor may bring new terminology standards (e.g., drug codes), content standards (e.g., clinical document formats), transport standards (e.g., imaging and communication protocols) and identifier standards (e.g. patient identifiers). The HIEs, thus, need to coordinate one-to-one connections between the new participant and the existing network each time. Another limitation of HIEs is that they do not provide any modern API.

In their simplest form, APIs act as software intermediaries between two or more applications. So, for example, each time a radiologist in healthcare provider A is checking patient imaging data that may have been stored in provider B and then communicating with other healthcare professionals across the HIEs, they are using API. The medical imaging application in healthcare provider A is connecting to the Internet and the application installed in the server of provider B to receive data. The server of healthcare provider A then retrieves that data, interprets it, performs the necessary actions and sends it to the radiologist's medical imaging application. The application then interprets that data and presents the radiologist with the information they wanted in a readable format. Most healthcare organizations today, including HIEs, use SOAP (simple object protocol) or RPC (remote procedural call protocol). SOAP is an API protocol that has been used since the 1990s, but comes with strict rules, rigid standards and is very resource intensive. Similarly, RPC is the oldest and simplest type of API protocol that is very tightly coupled to software architectures. In contrast, modern APIs are developed on REST (representational state transfer protocol), which drives most cloud-based applications today, from Netflix to Uber.

A second approach has the least impact of the three since it is primarily aimed at standardizing data across disparate information systems like EHRs within healthcare providers. Healthcare integration engines aim to improve workflows, optimize the delivery of care and streamline the integration and adoption of new technologies. This process involves the transformation of data between different standards and requires support for multiple transmission protocols. Although there are many commercial off-the-shelf integration engines such as Iguana and Rhapsody, these often allow message exchange using one standard and a small subset of transmission protocols. However, as discussed already, many technology providers use proprietary formats that are not compatible with formats designed by competing providers, and healthcare organizations will often develop custom point-to-point interface solutions that only aggravate the problem in the long run.[70] This approach does not provide any capabilities for scalable managed service across healthcare organizations.

A third approach currently being deployed by technology providers by means of addressing the interoperability challenge is EHR marketplaces. EHR systems were introduced as early as the 1970s with the objective of storing patient data, automating clinical workflows and supporting decision-making across operations within healthcare providers.[71] As discussed earlier, the variation in EHR systems across health organizations, including their custom integration with third-party applications or to in-house development has only aggravated interoperability challenges.[72]

In recent years, EHR technology providers, inspired by app marketplaces, have been motivated to develop EHR marketplaces. EHR marketplaces act as platforms that enable third-party developers to extend the capabilities of existing EHR systems through API and standards such as the FHIR (Fast Healthcare Interoperability Resources).[73] For example, the SMART (Substitutable Medical Applications, Reusable Technologies) App Gallery is an example of an EHR marketplace that enables a plug-and-play integration with participating EHRs.[74] The FHIR standard serves as the common data specification that both EHR provider APIs and SMART APIs adhere to. EHR marketplaces such as SMART increase open innovation while providing incentives for competition between app developers, including making their apps interoperable. Motivated by these benefits, some national governments like the Office of the National Coordinator for Health Information Technology in the USA require all providers to use HL7's FHIR Release 4 standard in their API by means of encouraging the development of apps that are interoperable.[75] Although these are welcome developments for addressing the interoperability challenge, open EHR marketplaces increase competition for technology providers without a clear governance framework with which to steer innovation and benefits for healthcare providers. Although FHIR is definitely a step forward from integration engines, the key challenge is that FHIR, just like other conventional approaches to solving the interoperability challenge, is organization-centric. However, to make the shift toward personalized medicine we need to deploy patient-centric models, with clinical workflows becoming the result of many intelligent decisions that do not stand alone, as separate, discreet and linear entities.[76]

This difference is often referred to as tethered vs untethered models for personal health records: whereas tethered models are "tightly connected to the system the provider uses to manage their organisation" such as a hospital, and are "often harder to make interoperable with other regional initiatives", untethered models "are standalone systems, provided by a health and care provider, or by an outside company"; they "give individuals control over who they share that data with, including health and care providers", and are "not restricted by the functionality of the organisation's internal system, such as an electronic medical record"; neither will they change "if the provider changes their internal system".[77] A great example of an untethered and integrated system is the Evergreen personal health record system that solves the interoperability challenge with the patient in the center.[78] Patients using the Evergreen Life app can receive information into their personal health record from different healthcare providers, while building a complete view of their health, including information they have recorded themselves. Patients can reuse data across other apps, can control which apps have access to their data and can reuse one set of user credentials across all their apps.

Unfortunately, most healthcare organizations rely on tethered – and often not with integrated – systems, thus suffering from the interoperability challenge. A lack of interoperability generates significant issues on data access which impede both the efficient management of the rising costs of healthcare services and doctor and carer burnout and the prevention of medical errors. Evidently, each of the challenges discussed in the previous sections is tightly interdependent on the technologies used in healthcare organizations and the data they use for their everyday clinical and administrative tasks. Data collected and exchanged through EHRs and other information systems and applications offer a window into clinical and administrative tasks, performance outcomes, including costs, and the effectiveness of care provided.

Accordingly, there are numerous challenges to achieving data quality.[79] Data quality can be defined as "the totality of features and characteristics of a data set, that bear on its ability to satisfy the needs that result from the intended use of the data".[80] Studies into the ways by which data from EHR systems are extracted for research or other purposes have revealed several types of data quality issues including deviation from standard or agreed-upon definitions, missing or omitted data, incorrectly entered data, data not entered into a searchable field, errors related to the structural or functional complexity of EHR systems and errors related to data migration issues, as well as cultural or organizational biases.[81]

First, data that is entered according to local definitions as opposed to internationally agreed definitions such as ICD codes lead to inconsistencies even within organizations and an inability to share them or aggregate them for analysis.[82] Second, data that was never added in the EHR system such as claims, data or doctor notes is often hard to recover afterward, especially as patients move between providers [83] Third, incorrectly entered data is probably the most common data quality issue and could lead to subsequent errors, especially when aggregating or searching for related data. Fourth, data is often entered inconsistently into one of several fields that are not searchable. Data is also often imported as text, especially in the case of doctor or administrator notes, which may serve the local instance of looking up notes for a specific patient, but they become unusable and not easily recovered by query when dealing with global instances of multiple patients. Fifth, and related to the fourth, many EHR systems have multiple places to enter the same data or may require a complex navigation to input the data. Such structural and functional complexity may add to data quality issues. Sixth, data migration issues may occur because of incompatible interfaces between systems and applications or because of human error. Finally, cultural and organizational biases on reporting different conditions such as obesity[84] may introduce further issues on data quality. Correcting systemic issues in data quality is much easier at the point of data entry than at the point of data analysis or subsequent use by healthcare professionals within providers or across other organizations. The quality of the input data will dictate the quality of the output or as the axiom goes: "garbage in garbage out".

As healthcare organizations are moving toward digital transformation, being able to identify issues of data quality and understand their interdependencies to the challenges in healthcare service provision becomes a strategic priority.

2.4   The Ethical and Regulatory Challenges of Governing Data

Digital transformation is critical for addressing many of the challenges discussed in the previous sections. Such transformation in healthcare service provision is happening across multiple dimensions. From new prevention techniques and cures through to new vaccines and immunotherapy, as well as innovation in medical devices, medical imaging and diagnostics, and new applications of AI, blockchain infrastructures and cloud computing, healthcare is being transformed (Chapters 5–7 cover many of these digital innovations).

These transformations are increasingly data-driven and have the potential to reorder the relationships among – and processes between – healthcare providers, medical equipment manufacturers, patients, governments, public research, insurance companies and other ecosystem actors. The convergence of digital and biological technologies is disrupting healthcare and increasing the importance of interoperability and data integration across healthcare organizations. Despite these benefits, to achieve such transformation several ethical and regulatory challenges will have to be addressed.[85]

First, the privacy and security of patient and other types of data becomes a critical challenge. Regulations such as HIPAA in the USA and GDPR in Europe legally oblige healthcare service providers to protect their data, most importantly, the data of their patients, and to notify relevant parties about data breaches. Although healthcare service providers outsource some security controls to a cloud provider, they cannot outsource their responsibility for protecting their own data. Many healthcare service providers do not know where the cloud provider's responsibility for security controls starts and where it ends. This is exploited by cloud providers who often refuse to take responsibility for implementing particular security controls. Unfortunately, ambiguity over security controls can lead to security vulnerabilities that put patient data at risk. This challenge becomes even more prominent when cloud providers transfer data across regional and national borders, where little consensus exists about which authorities have jurisdiction over the data.[86]

There is growing awareness around the inequalities in technology and data access, as well as the control over those.[87] Recent scandals, like the case of Google DeepMind and the Royal Free London NHS Foundation Trust, which led to the transfer of identifiable patient records across the entire Trust without explicit consent are cases to remind us of the challenge of keeping data safe.[88] DeepMind was contracted to build a smartphone app, called 'Streams', to help clinicians manage acute kidney injury (AKI) linked to 40,000 deaths a year in the UK. Although the data that DeepMind was supposed to process under the Royal Free project were only limited to patients being monitored by clinicians for AKI, the actual dataset transferred to DeepMind extended much more broadly than this. In fact, it included every patient admission, discharge and transfer within the hospitals of Royal Free over a five-year period. Google eventually released a statement that this data was not just being used for the smartphone app, but also being shared for the development of real-time analysis and alert systems, potentially as part of a broadly defined "analytics as a service" platform. Cases like these lead to calls for greater regulation of health data, as those are being accessed and shared by various organizations through such technologies as AI. Clearly, many forms of data can be considered sensitive, where their abuse or misuse could result in harm to the individual concerned, from patients, to doctors, to insurance agents and many more.

Regulations such as the GDPR cover a wider set of data types than have previously been the case with data protection legislation. However, the sheer size of the datasets used in data-driven technologies, including AI technologies for medical, administrative or other use, makes such regulation potentially impractical – it may be impossible to get informed consent from each data consumer (e.g., a patient) or data custodian (e.g., a health provider) whose data is in a particular training dataset. Although anonymized, historical data can be retrospectively used for research without seeking specific consent, thus, prospective data use is challenging. For example, it is impossible to state, at the point of collection, exactly how an algorithm will use a particular data point and whether this will be important for the algorithm in the process of analysis. In other words, it is impossible to identify which data will be important for a specific use upfront. This means that data governance frameworks may need to be developed and tested that bypass informed consent as a legal and ethical basis on which to conduct data collection for use in different technologies.[89] The National Data Opt-Out program, which is being run by NHS Digital in the UK, is one such framework. Under this program, patients and the public who decide they do not want their personally identifiable data to be used for planning and research purposes will be able to set their national data opt-out choice online or via a "non-digital alternative".[90]

Yet, opt-out initiatives, as well as deliberate efforts by data custodians to de-identify data when opting-in (i.e., HIPAA compliance), are still not fully protected by data breaches and aggregation of information into large datasets that increases the potential for patient data being used in ways patients never would have intended. Although the illegitimate use of health data is now largely limited, the sophistication of big data use by commercial entities suggests that this concern is not unfounded.[91] For example, a recent study by the *Financial Times*[92] analyzed 100 health websites, including WebMD, Healthline, health insurance group Bupa and parenting site Babycentre, only to find that 79 percent of them dropped cookies on visitors, allowing them to be tracked by third-party companies around the Internet. The data included medical diagnoses, symptoms, prescriptions and menstrual and fertility information. This was done without consent, making the practice illegal under GDPR. By far the most common destination for the data was Google's advertising arm DoubleClick, which showed up in 78 percent of the sites the *Financial Times* had tested. This sort of rampant rule-breaking has been a known loophole in the advertising industry, which is worth $615 billion globally.[93]

Such illegitimate uses of health data are not contained in advertising. There are growing concerns of the very real risks of discrimination based on health data in health insurance, life insurance, and employment based on pre-existing health conditions. Data discrimination results in practices that exclude segments of the population from access to healthcare services. For example, recent advances in genetic testing to predict many different individual characteristics and phenotypes including the propensity for disease have given rise to concerns about genetic discrimination in employment, life and health insurance.[94] Most countries have already established regulation that prohibits genetic discrimination from the *Convention on Biomedicine* (1997) and the *Charter of Fundamental Rights of the European Union* (2000), to the *Genetic Information Nondiscrimination Act* (2008) in the USA (2008), the *Concordat and Moratorium on Genetics and Insurance* in the UK and the Australian *Disability Discrimination Act* (2008). However, these regulations hardly address the complex ways by which data are pried upon. For example, individual data can be tracked and monitored through productivity apps, personal devices and wearables such as mobile phones and smart watches, and social media profiles and credit reports.[95] Genetic data is arguably harder to get hold of, but as the example of Babycentre mentioned above shows, often genetic data is accessed indirectly through third parties.

Another challenge that is closely associated to data discrimination is data bias "that is, the use of datasets that are not fully representative of the population they seek to typify".[96] Recent reports have argued that most often bias is built into the technologies we use, but also in the very ways by which the tech industry works from a dire lack of diversity among employees to damaging discrimination in the algorithms embedded in AI systems including sex, race, ethnicity or ability.[97] Increasing the diversity of experience in tech employees is a fundamental requirement for those who develop new digital technologies in an effort to identify and reduce the harms those technologies produce.[98]

New digital innovations including AI, Internet of Things (IoT) devices and cloud-computing have made it possible to classify and analyze large amounts of data, allowing technology companies to monitor everyday experiences like going for a walk, food shopping, sleeping and menstruating to predicting people's health behavior and medical condition.[99] While such developments may offer future positive health benefits, these innovations have challenged the boundaries of healthcare services. The scope and scale of these new "algorithmic health infrastructures"[100] give rise to several ethical and regulatory concerns. Technology companies often make lucrative data partnership agreements with a wide range of healthcare organizations to gain access to health data for the training and development of new digital technologies. The potential misuse of these new digital technologies could impact healthcare access or stigmatize individuals such as recent attempts to diagnose complex mental health conditions from social-media data.[101] There are possible social harms for patients such as the potential for clinical decisions to be nudged or guided by digital technologies in ways that do not bring about health benefits but are in service for performance requirements or increased profit. Importantly, misuses also extend beyond the ethics of patient care to consider how digital technologies are reshaping medical organizations themselves (e.g., radiologist and radiology departments will also be data for healthcare administrators) and the wider health domain by blurring the line between academic research and commercial uses of health data.[102] Even when designed with good intentions new digital technologies may end up worsening health inequities.[103]

These ethical and regulatory challenges will always be present as new advances in digital, biogenetic and other types of technologies continue to be introduced into healthcare services. They can, however, be mitigated when hospitals, insurers, patients and regulators start to cooperate more closely to influence the rate and direction of innovation while accommodating diverse needs. For this to materialize, these actors will have to create and use digital technologies to exchange relevant information and feedback, while specifying targets and focus areas and by helping to align the costs and benefits of innovation. The next chapters explore how organization and digital transformation can be achieved across healthcare ecosystems.

Notes

1 Mossialos, E., Dixon, A., Figueras, J., and Kutzin, J., eds. 2002. *Funding Health Care: Options for Europe*. Open University Press, London UK; Pauly, M., McGuire, T., Barros, P., eds. 2012. *Handbook of Health Economics, Vol. 2*. Elsevier, Amsterdam, The Netherlands; see also *China's Yearbook on Health and Family Planning* https://www.chinayearbooks.com/chinas-health-and-family-planning-statistical-yearbook-2016.html

2 WHO. 2019. Global Spending on Health: A World in Transition https://www.who.int/health_financing/documents/health-expenditure-report-2019/en/

3 Gómez-Aguado, I., Rodríguez-Castejón, J., Vicente-Pascual, M., Rodríguez-Gascón, A., Solinís, M.Á. and del Pozo-Rodríguez, A., 2020. Nanomedicines to deliver mRNA: state of the art and future perspectives. *Nanomaterials*, 10(2), p. 364; Lin, Y.X., Wang, Y., Blake, S., Yu, M., Mei, L., Wang, H. and Shi, J., 2020. RNA nanotechnology-mediated cancer immunotherapy. *Theranostics*, 10(1), p. 281.

4 Legorreta, A.P., Silber, J.H., Costantino, G.N., Kobylinski, R.W. and Zatz, S.L., 1993. Increased cholecystectomy rate after the introduction of laparoscopic cholecystectomy. *Jama*, 270(12), pp. 1429–1432; Chernew, M., Fendrick, A.M. and Hirth, R.A., 1997. Managed care and medical technology: implications for cost growth. *Health Affairs*, 16(2), pp. 196–206.

5 Gupta, V. and Jain, G., 2019. Safe laparoscopic cholecystectomy: adoption of universal culture of safety in cholecystectomy. *World Journal of Gastrointestinal Surgery*, 11(2), p. 62; Conrad, C., Wakabayashi, G., Asbun, H.J., Dallemagne, B., Demartines, N., Diana, M., Fuks, D., Giménez, M.E., Goumard, C., Kaneko, H. and Memeo, R., 2017. IRCAD recommendation on safe laparoscopic cholecystectomy. *Journal of Hepato-Biliary-Pancreatic Sciences*, 24(11), pp. 603–615; Barrett, M., Asbun, H.J., Chien, H.L., Brunt, L.M. and Telem, D.A., 2018. Bile duct injury and morbidity following cholecystectomy: a need for improvement. *Surgical Endoscopy*, 32(4), pp. 1683–1688.

6 Berndt, E.R., McGuire, T.G. and Newhouse, J.P., 2011. A primer on the economics of prescription pharmaceutical pricing in health insurance markets. NBER Working Paper 16879.

7 Garber, A.M., Jones, C.I. and Romer, P., 2006. Insurance and incentives for medical innovation. *Forum for Health Economics & Policy*, 9(2) (Article 4).

8 Pauly, M., McGuire, T., Barros, P., eds. 2012. *Handbook of Health Economics, Vol. 2*. Elsevier, Amsterdam, The Netherlands

9 See the definition of QUALY provided by NICE https://www.nice.org.uk/glossary?letter=q

10 Whitehead, S.J. and Ali, S., 2010. Health outcomes in economic evaluation: the QALY and utilities. *British Medical Bulletin*, 96(1), pp. 5–21.

11 Dolan, P. and Kahneman, D., 2008. Interpretations of utility and their implications for the valuation of health. *The Economic Journal*, 118(525), pp. 215–234.

12 Mathews, A.W., 2018. Behind your rising health-care bills: secret hospital deals that squelch competition, *Wall Street Journal*, September 22, 2018.

13 Makary, M., 2019. *The Price We Pay: What Broke American Health Care – and How to Fix it*. Bloomsbury Publishing, New York USA.

14 Kliff, S., Katz, J. and Taylor, R., 2021. Hospitals and Insurers didn't want you to see these prices. Here's Why. *NYT Online* https://www.nytimes.com/interactive/2021/08/22/upshot/hospital-prices.html

15 Ibid.

16 Grieve, R., Hutton, J., Bhalla, A., Rastenyte, D., Ryglewicz, D., Sarti, C., Lamassa, M., Giroud, M., Dundas, R. and Wolfe, C.D.A., 2001. A comparison of the costs and survival of hospital-admitted stroke patients across Europe. *Stroke*, 32(7), pp. 1684–1691.

17 Wei, J.W., Heeley, E.L., Jan, S., Huang, Y., Huang, Q., Wang, J.G., Cheng, Y., Xu, E., Yang, Q., Anderson, C.S. and ChinaQUEST Investigators, 2010. Variations and determinants of hospital costs for acute stroke in China. *PloS One*, 5(9), p. e13041.

18 See https://www.choosingwisely.org/ and the original study that led to this initiative: Cassel, C.K. and Guest, J.A., 2012. Choosing wisely: helping physicians and patients make smart decisions about their care. *JAMA*, 307(17), pp. 1801–1802.

19 Colla, C.H., Morden, N.E., Sequist, T.D., Schpero, W.L. and Rosenthal, M.B., 2015. Choosing wisely: prevalence and correlates of low-value health care services in the United States. *Journal of General Internal Medicine*, 30(2), pp. 221–228.

20 Ibid.

21 Mason, D.J., 2015. Choosing wisely: changing clinicians, patients, or policies? *JAMA*, 313(7), pp. 657–658.

22 Selden, T.M., Karaca, Z., Keenan, P., White, C. and Kronick, R., 2015. The growing difference between public and private payment rates for inpatient hospital care. *Health Affairs*, 34(12), pp. 2147–2150; White, C. and Whaley, C., 2019. Prices paid to hospitals by private health plans are high relative to Medicare and vary widely. Santa Monica, CA: Rand Corporation https://www.rand.org/pubs/research_reports/RR3033.html.

23 Welch, H.G., Prorok, P.C., O'Malley, A.J. and Kramer, B.S., 2016. Breast-cancer tumor size, overdiagnosis, and mammography screening effectiveness. *The New England Journal of Medicine*, 375(15), pp. 1438–1447.

24 Pinsky, P.F., Prorok, P.C. and Kramer, B.S., 2017. Prostate cancer screening—a perspective on the current state of the evidence. *The New England Journal of Medicine*, 376(13), pp. 1285–1289.

25 Timmermans, S. and Berg, M., 2010. *The Gold Standard: The Challenge of Evidence-Based Medicine*. Temple University Press, Philadelphia, USA

26 Maslach, C. and Leiter, M.P., 2016. Understanding the burnout experience: recent research and its implications for psychiatry. *World Psychiatry*, 15(2), pp. 103–111.

27 De Hert, S., 2020. Burnout in healthcare workers: prevalence, impact and preventative strategies. *Local and Regional Anesthesia*, 13, p. 171; Pavelková, H. and Bužgová, R., 2015. Burnout among healthcare workers in hospice care. *Central European Journal of Nursing and Midwifery*, 6(1), pp. 218–223; Embriaco, N., Papazian, L., Kentish-Barnes, N., Pochard, F. and Azoulay, E., 2007. Burnout syndrome among critical care healthcare workers. *Current Opinion in Critical Care*, 13(5), pp. 482–488; Peterson, U., Demerouti, E., Bergström, G., Samuelsson, M., Åsberg, M. and Nygren, Å., 2008. Burnout and physical and mental health among Swedish healthcare workers. *Journal of Advanced Nursing*, 62(1), pp. 84–95.

28 Medscape National Physician Burnout & Suicide Report 2020. Available from: https://www.medscape.com/slideshow/2020-lifestyle-burnout-6012460.

29 Embriaco, N., Papazian, L., Kentish-Barnes, N., Pochard, F. and Azoulay, E., 2007. Burnout syndrome among critical care healthcare workers. *Current Opinion in Critical Care*, 13(5), pp. 482–488; Peterson, U., Demerouti, E., Bergström, G., Samuelsson, M., Åsberg, M. and Nygren, Å., 2008. Burnout and physical and mental health among Swedish healthcare workers. *Journal of Advanced Nursing*, 62(1), pp. 84–95.

30 Dyrbye, L.N., West, C.P., Satele, D., Boone, S., Tan, L., Sloan, J. and Shanafelt, T.D., 2014. Burnout among US medical students, residents, and early career physicians relative to the general US population. *Academic Medicine*, 89(3), pp. 443–451.

31 Soler, J.K., Yaman, H., Esteva, M., Dobbs, F., Asenova, R.S., Katić, M., Ožvačić, Z., Desgranges, J.P., Moreau, A., Lionis, C. and Kotányi, P., 2008. Burnout in European family doctors: the EGPRN study. *Family Practice*, 25(4), pp. 245–265.

32 Imo, U.O., 2017. Burnout and psychiatric morbidity among doctors in the UK: a systematic literature review of prevalence and associated factors. *BJPsych Bulletin*, 41(4), pp. 197–204.

33 Chemali, Z., Ezzeddine, F.L., Gelaye, B., Dossett, M.L., Salameh, J., Bizri, M., Dubale, B. and Fricchione, G., 2019. Burnout among healthcare providers in the complex environment of the Middle East: a systematic review. *BMC Public Health*, 19(1), pp. 1–21.

34 Dyrbye, L. and Shanafelt, T., 2016. A narrative review on burnout experienced by medical students and residents. *Medical Education*, 50(1), pp. 132–149.

35 Perez, H.R., Beyrouty, M., Bennett, K., Manwell, L.B., Brown, R.L., Linzer, M. and Schwartz, M.D., 2017. Chaos in the clinic: characteristics and consequences of practices perceived as chaotic. *The Journal for Healthcare Quality (JHQ)*, 39(1), pp. 43–53.

36 Haque, M., Sartelli, M., McKimm, J. and Bakar, M.A., 2018. Health care-associated infections – an overview. *Infection and Drug Resistance*, 11, p. 2321; Restrepo, D., Armstrong, K.A. and Metlay, J.P., 2020. Annals clinical decision making: avoiding cognitive errors in clinical decision making. *Annals of Internal Medicine*, 172(11), pp. 747–751; Kane-Gill, S.L., Dasta, J.F., Buckley, M.S., Devabhakthuni, S., Liu, M., Cohen, H., George, E.L., Pohlman, A.S., Agarwal, S., Henneman, E.A. and Bejian, S.M., 2017. Clinical practice guideline: safe medication use in the ICU. *Critical Care Medicine*, 45(9), pp. e877–e915; Hammoudi, B.M., Ismaile, S. and Abu Yahya, O., 2018. Factors associated with medication administration errors and why nurses fail to report them. *Scandinavian Journal of Caring Sciences*, 32(3), pp. 1038–1046.

37 DeVine, J., Chutkan, N., Norvell, D.C. and Dettori, J.R., 2010. Avoiding wrong site surgery: a systematic review. *Spine*, 35(9 S), pp. S28–S36; Stahel, P.F., Sabel, A.L., Victoroff, M.S., Varnell, J., Lembitz, A., Boyle, D.J., Clarke, T.J., Smith, W.R. and Mehler, P.S., 2010. Wrong-site and wrong-patient procedures in the universal protocol era: analysis of a prospective database of physician self-reported occurrences. *Archives of Surgery*, 145(10), pp. 978–984.

38 Griffen, F.D., Stephens, L.S., Alexander, J.B., Bailey, H.R., Maizel, S.E., Sutton, B.H. and Posner, K.L., 2007. The American College of Surgeons' closed claims study: new insights for improving care. *Journal of the American College of Surgeons*, 204(4), pp. 561–569; Shanafelt, T.D., Balch, C.M., Bechamps, G., Russell, T., Dyrbye, L., Satele, D., Collicott, P., Novotny, P.J., Sloan, J. and Freischlag, J., 2010. Burnout and medical errors among American surgeons. *Annals of Surgery*, 251(6), pp. 995–1000.

39 Regenbogen, S.E., Greenberg, C.C., Studdert, D.M., Lipsitz, S.R., Zinner, M.J. and Gawande, A.A., 2007. Patterns of technical error among surgical malpractice claims: an analysis of strategies to prevent injury to surgical patients. *Annals of Surgery*, 246(5), pp. 705–711; Jena, A.B., Schoemaker, L., Bhattacharya, J. and Seabury, S.A., 2015. Physician spending and subsequent risk of malpractice claims: observational study. *BMJ 351*, h5516.

40 Robertson, J.J. and Long, B., 2018. Suffering in silence: medical error and its impact on health care providers. *The Journal of Emergency Medicine*, 54(4), pp.402–409; Ozeke, O., Ozeke, V., Coskun, O. and Budakoglu, I.I., 2019. Second victims in health care: current perspectives. *Advances in Medical Education and Practice*, 10, p. 593.

41 Lucas, B.P., Trick, W.E., Evans, A.T., Mba, B., Smith, J., Das, K., Clarke, P., Varkey, A., Mathew, S. and Weinstein, R.A., 2012. Effects of 2-vs 4-week attending physician inpatient rotations on unplanned patient revisits, evaluations by trainees, and attending physician burnout: a randomized trial. *JAMA*, 308(21), pp. 2199–2207.

42 Linzer, M., Poplau, S., Grossman, E., Varkey, A., Yale, S., Williams, E., Hicks, L., Brown, R.L., Wallock, J., Kohnhorst, D. and Barbouche, M., 2015. A cluster randomized trial of interventions to improve work conditions and clinician burnout in primary care: results from the Healthy Work Place (HWP) study. *Journal of General Internal Medicine*, 30(8), pp. 1105–1111.

43 Parshuram, C.S., Amaral, A.C., Ferguson, N.D., Baker, G.R., Etchells, E.E., Flintoft, V., Granton, J., Lingard, L., Kirpalani, H., Mehta, S. and Moldofsky, H., 2015. Patient safety, resident well-being and continuity of care with different resident duty schedules in the intensive care unit: a randomized trial. *Cmaj*, 187(5), pp. 321–329.

44 West, C.P., Dyrbye, L.N., Rabatin, J.T., Call, T.G., Davidson, J.H., Multari, A., Romanski, S.A., Hellyer, J.M.H., Sloan, J.A. and Shanafelt, T.D., 2014. Intervention to promote physician well-being, job satisfaction, and professionalism: a randomized clinical trial. *JAMA Internal Medicine*, 174(4), pp. 527–533.

45 Moody, K., Kramer, D., Santizo, R.O., Magro, L., Wyshogrod, D., Ambrosio, J., Castillo, C., Lieberman, R. and Stein, J., 2013. Helping the helpers: mindfulness training for burnout in pediatric oncology – a pilot program. *Journal of Pediatric Oncology Nursing*, 30(5), pp. 275–284.

46 Bragard, I., Etienne, A.M., Merckaert, I., Libert, Y. and Razavi, D., 2010. Efficacy of a communication and stress management training on medical residents' self-efficacy, stress to communicate and burnout: a randomized controlled study. *Journal of Health Psychology*, 15(7), pp. 1075–1081.

47 Jensen, P.M., Trollope-Kumar, K., Waters, H. and Everson, J., 2008. Building physician resilience. *Canadian Family Physician*, 54(5), pp. 722–729.

48 Shanafelt, T.D., Balch, C.M., Bechamps, G., Russell, T., Dyrbye, L., Satele, D., Collicott, P., Novotny, P.J., Sloan, J. and Freischlag, J., 2010. Burnout and medical errors among American surgeons. *Annals of Surgery*, 251(6), pp. 995–1000.

49 Petersen, L.A., Woodard, L.D., Urech, T., Daw, C. and Sookanan, S., 2006. Does pay-for-performance improve the quality of health care?. *Annals of Internal Medicine*, 145(4), pp. 265–272.

50 Cerasoli, C.P., Nicklin, J.M. and Ford, M.T., 2014. Intrinsic motivation and extrinsic incentives jointly predict performance: a 40-year meta-analysis. *Psychological Bulletin*, 140(4), p. 980.

51 Weibel, A., Rost, K. and Osterloh, M., 2010. Pay for performance in the public sector – benefits and (hidden) costs. *Journal of Public Administration Research and Theory*, 20(2), pp. 387–412; Petersen, L.A., Woodard, L.D., Urech, T., Daw, C. and Sookanan, S., 2006. Does pay-for-performance improve the quality of health care?. *Annals of Internal Medicine*, 145(4), pp. 265–272.

52 Cooper, M.D., 2000. Towards a model of safety culture. *Safety Science*, 36(2), pp. 111–136; Guldenmund, F.W., 2000. The nature of safety culture: a review of theory and research. *Safety Science*, 34(1–3), pp. 215–257; Leape, L., Berwick, D., Clancy, C., Conway, J., Gluck, P., Guest, J., Lawrence, D., Morath, J., O'Leary, D., O'Neill, P. and Pinakiewicz, D., 2009. Transforming healthcare: a safety imperative. *BMJ Quality & Safety*, 18(6), pp. 424–428; Weaver, S.J., Lubomksi, L.H., Wilson, R.F., Pfoh, E.R., Martinez, K.A. and Dy, S.M., 2013. Promoting a culture of safety as a patient safety strategy: a systematic review. *Annals of Internal Medicine*, 158(5_Part_2), pp. 369–374.

53 Weaver, S.J., Lubomksi, L.H., Wilson, R.F., Pfoh, E.R., Martinez, K.A. and Dy, S.M., 2013. Promoting a culture of safety as a patient safety strategy: a systematic review. *Annals of Internal Medicine*, 158(5_Part_2), pp. 369–374.

54 Leape, L., Berwick, D., Clancy, C., Conway, J., Gluck, P., Guest, J., Lawrence, D., Morath, J., O'Leary, D., O'Neill, P. and Pinakiewicz, D., 2009. Transforming healthcare: a safety imperative. *BMJ Quality & Safety*, 18(6), pp. 424–428

55 Cooper, M.D., 2000. Towards a model of safety culture. *Safety Science*, 36(2), pp. 111–136.

56 https://www.statista.com/statistics/1037970/global-healthcare-data-volume/

57 Topol, E.J., 2014. Individualized medicine from prewomb to tomb. *Cell*, 157(1), pp. 241–253.

58 Constantinides, P. (ed.), 2012. *Perspectives and Implications for the Development of Information Infrastructures*. IGI Global, Hershey, USA; European Commission. 1994. *Europe's Way to the Information Society: An Action Plan*. Brussels: European Commission; Department of Health (DoH). 2002. *Delivering 21st century IT Support for the NHS – National Strategic Programme*. Department of Health, UK; Advisory Committee on Health Infostructure (ACHI). 2001. Tactical plan for a pan-Canadian health infostructure, 2001 update. Office of Health and the Information Highway, Health Canada; National Committee on Vital and Health Statistics (NCVHS). 2001. *Information for Health: A Strategy for Building the National Health Information Infrastructure*. Washington: U.S. Department of Health and Human Services; NHIMAC. 2001. Health online: a health information action plan for Australia. National Health Information Management Advisory Council, Australian Institute of Health and Welfare. 2nd edition, September 2001; World Health Organization, 2012. *National eHealth Strategy Toolkit*. International Telecommunication Union, Geneva, Switzerland

59 WHO, 2008. Building foundations eHealth in Europe: Report of the WHO Global Observatory for eHealth. World Health Organization [online] Available at: http://www.who.int/goe/BFeuroFull.pdf

60 HIMSS https://www.himss.org/resources/interoperability-healthcare; COCIR, 2013. E-health toolkit healthcare transformation towards seamless integrated care. 3rd edition. COCIR. Available at: http://www.cocir.org/fileadmin/Publications_2013/COCIR_eHealth_Toolkit_2013.pdf

61 Constantinides, P., 2013. The communicative constitution of IT innovation. *Information and Organization*, 23(4), pp. 215–232.

62 Department of Health (DoH). 2002. *Delivering 21st century IT support for the NHS – national strategic programme*. UK: Department of Health.

63 Justinia, T., 2017. The UK's National Programme for IT: Why was it dismantled?. *Health Services Management Research*, 30(1), pp. 2–9.

64 Hays, G. M., Shepherd, I., Humphries, R., Beer, G., Carpenter, G. I., Asbridge, J., et al. (2009). *Independent Review of NHS and Social Care IT.* Commissioned by Stephen O'Brien, Conservative member of Parliament.

65 Coiera, E., 2009. Building a national health IT system from the middle out. *Journal of the American Medical Informatics Association,* 16(3), pp. 271–273; Yang, Z., Ng, B.Y., Kankanhalli, A. and Yip, J.W.L., 2012. Workarounds in the use of IS in healthcare: a case study of an electronic medication administration system. *International Journal of Human-Computer Studies,* 70(1), pp. 43–65; Vogelsmeier, A.A., Halbesleben, J.R. and Scott-Cawiezell, J.R., 2008. Technology implementation and workarounds in the nursing home. *Journal of the American Medical Informatics Association,* 15(1), pp. 114–119.

66 Dixon, B., 2016. Health information exchange (HIE): navigating and managing a network of health information systems, in *Health Information Exchange (HIE): Navigating and Managing a Network of Health Information Systems.* Elsevier Academic Press, Amsterdam, The Netherlands; Vest, J.R. and Gamm, L.D., 2010. Health information exchange: persistent challenges and new strategies. *Journal of the American Medical Informatics Association,* 17(3), pp. 288–294; Kuperman, G.J., 2011. Health-information exchange: why are we doing it, and what are we doing?. *Journal of the American Medical Informatics Association,* 18(5), pp. 678–682; Constantinides, P. and Barrett, M., 2006. Large-scale ICT innovation, power, and organizational change: the case of a regional health information network. *The Journal of Applied Behavioral Science,* 42(1), pp. 76–90.

67 Adler-Milstein, J., McAfee, A. P., Bates, D.W. and Jha, A.K., 2008. The state of regional health information organizations: current activities and financing. *Health Affairs,* 27(1), pp. 60–69; Braa, J., Monteiro, E. and Sahay, S., 2004. Networks of action: sustainable health information systems across developing countries. *MIS Quarterly,* 28(3), pp. 337–362; Sahay, S., Monteiro, E. and Aanestad, M., 2009. Configurable politics and asymmetric integration: health e-infrastructures in India. *Journal of the Association for Information Systems,* 10(5), pp. 399–414; Cho, S. and Mathiassen, L., 2007. The role of industry infrastructure in tele-health innovations: a multi-level analysis of a telestroke program. *European Journal of Information Systems,* 16(6), pp. 738–750; Constantinides, P. and Barrett, M., 2015. Information infrastructure development and governance as collective action. *Information Systems Research,* 26(1), pp. 40–56; Jensen, T.B. and Aanestad, M., 2007. Hospitality and hostility in hospitals: a case study of an EPR adoption among surgeons. *European Journal of Information Systems,* 16(6), pp. 672–680.

68 Coiera, E., 2009. Building a national health IT system from the middle out. Journalof the American Medical Informatics Association, 16(3), pp. 271–273.

69 Dixon, B., 2016. Health information exchange (HIE): navigating and managing a network of health information systems. *Health Information Exchange (HIE): Navigating and Managing a Network of Health Information Systems.* Academic Press.

70 Bortis, G., 2008. Experiences with Mirth: an open source health care integration engine. In *Proceedings of the 30th International Conference on Software Engineering,* pp. 649–652.

71 Gillum, R.F., 2013. From papyrus to the electronic tablet: a brief history of the clinical medical record with lessons for the digital age. *The American Journal of Medicine,* 126(10), pp. 853–857.

72 Ludwick, D.A. and Doucette, J., 2009. Adopting electronic medical records in primary care: lessons learned from health information systems implementation experience in seven countries. *International Journal of Medical Informatics,* 78(1), pp. 22–31.

73 Sittig, D.F. and Wright, A., 2015. What makes an EHR "open" or interoperable?. *Journal of the American Medical Informatics Association,* 22(5), pp. 1099–1101.

74 Mandel, J.C., Kreda, D.A., Mandl, K.D., Kohane, I.S. and Ramoni, R.B., 2016. SMART on FHIR: a standards-based, interoperable apps platform for electronic health records. *Journal of the American Medical Informatics Association,* 23(5), pp. 899–908.

75 See the ONC's 21st Century Cures Act here https://www.healthit.gov/curesrule/what-it-means-for-me/health-it-developers

76 I thank Stephen Critchlow, Founder, CEO and Chair of the Wellbeing Team at Evergreen Life for helping me understand the point of shifting from an organizational to a patient-centric model.

77 https://digital.nhs.uk/services/personal-health-records-adoption-service/personal-health-records-adoption-toolkit/developing-a-personal-health-record/technical-architectures-for-personal-health-records

78 https://www.evergreen-life.co.uk/evergreen-life-app/

79 Weiskopf, N.G. and Weng, C., 2013. Methods and dimensions of electronic health record data quality assessment: enabling reuse for clinical research. *Journal of the American Medical Informatics Association*, 20(1), pp. 144–151; Arts, D.G., De Keizer, N.F. and Scheffer, G.J., 2002. Defining and improving data quality in medical registries: a literature review, case study, and generic framework. *Journal of the American Medical Informatics Association*, 9(6), pp. 600–611.

80 Arts, D.G., De Keizer, N.F. and Scheffer, G.J., 2002. Defining and improving data quality in medical registries: a literature review, case study, and generic framework. *Journal of the American Medical Informatics Association*, 9(6), pp. 600–611. This definition is closely aligned with the International Standards Organization (ISO) 8000–8:2015 definition of data quality https://www.iso.org/standard/60805.html. This definition incorporates three parts: "*syntactic quality*, which is the degree to which data conforms to its specified syntax, i.e. requirements stated by the metadata; *semantic quality*, which is the degree to which data corresponds to what it represents; *pragmatic quality*, which is the degree to which data is found suitable and worthwhile for a particular purpose".

81 Hartzband, D. and Jacobs, F., 2016. Deployment of analytics into the healthcare safety net: Lessons learned. *Online Journal of Public Health Informatics*, 8(3), pp. 1–13; Kahn, M.G., Raebel, M.A., Glanz, J.M., Riedlinger, K. and Steiner, J.F., 2012. A pragmatic framework for single-site and multisite data quality assessment in electronic health record-based clinical research. *Medical Care*, 50, pp. 1–16.

82 O'malley, K.J., Cook, K.F., Price, M.D., Wildes, K.R., Hurdle, J.F. and Ashton, C.M., 2005. Measuring diagnoses: ICD code accuracy. *Health Services Research*, 40(5p2), pp. 1620–1639; Rollason, W., Khunti, K. and De Lusignan, S., 2009. Variation in the recording of diabetes diagnostic data in primary care computer systems: implications for the quality of care. *Journal of Innovation in Health Informatics*, 17(2), pp. 113–119.

83 DeVoe, J.E., Gold, R., McIntire, P., Puro, J., Chauvie, S. and Gallia, C.A., 2011. Electronic health records vs Medicaid claims: completeness of diabetes preventive care data in community health centers. *The Annals of Family Medicine*, 9(4), pp. 351–358.

84 Al Kazzi, E.S., Lau, B., Li, T., Schneider, E.B., Makary, M.A. and Hutfless, S., 2015. Differences in the prevalence of obesity, smoking and alcohol in the United States nationwide inpatient sample and the behavioral risk factor surveillance system. *PLoS One*, 10(11), p.e0140165.

85 Metcalfe, J. S., James, A. and Mina, A., 2005. Emergent innovation systems and the delivery of clinical services: the case of intra-ocular lenses. *Research Policy*, 34(9), pp. 1283–1304; Herzlinger, R. E. (2006). Why innovation in health care Is so hard. *Harvard Business Review*, 84(5), pp. 58–66.

86 Seddon, J.J. and Currie, W.L., 2013. Cloud computing and trans-border health data: unpacking US and EU healthcare regulation and compliance. *Health Policy and Technology*, 2(4), pp. 229–241.

87 Weiss, D., Rydland, H.T., Øversveen, E., Jensen, M.R., Solhaug, S. and Krokstad, S., 2018. Innovative technologies and social inequalities in health: a scoping review of the literature. *PloS One*, 13(4), p. e0195447; Venkatesh, V., Rai, A., Sykes, T.A., and Aljafari, R., 2016. Combating infant mortality in rural India: evidence from a field study of EHealth Kiosk implementations. *MIS Quarterly*, 40(2), pp. 353–380; Downing, N.S., Shah, N.D., Neiman, J.H., Aminawung, J.A., Krumholz, H.M., and Ross, J.S., 2016. Participation of the elderly, women, and minorities in pivotal trials supporting 2011–2013 U.S. Food and Drug Administration approvals. *Trials*, 17(1), p. 199.

88 Powles, J. and Hodson, H., 2017. Google DeepMind and healthcare in an age of algorithms. *Health and Technology*, 7(4), pp. 351–367.

89 Future Advocacy. 2018. *Ethical, Social, and Political Challenges of Artificial Intelligence in Health*. A report with The Wellcome Trust. April 11, 2018. https://futureadvocacy.com/publications/ethical-social-and-political-challenges-of-artificial-intelligence-in-health/

90 See the Academy of Medical Sciences' Understanding Patient Data Project https://acmedsci. ac.uk/policy/policy-projects/use-of-patient-data-in-healthcare-and-research

91 Cassel, C., and Bindman, A., 2019. Risk, benefit, and fairness in a big data world. *JAMA, 322*(2), pp. 105–106; Bardhan, I., Chen, H. and Karahanna, E., 2020. Connecting systems, data, and people: a multidisciplinary research roadmap for chronic disease management. *MIS Quarterly, 44*(1), pp. 185–200.

92 FT investigation into how top health websites are sharing sensitive data with advertisers https://www.ft.com/content/0fbf4d8e-022b-11ea-be59-e49b2a136b8d

93 https://www.researchandmarkets.com/reports/5769211/global-advertising-market-industry-trends

94 Chapman, C.R., Mehta, K.S., Parent, B. and Caplan, A.L., 2020. Genetic discrimination: emerging ethical challenges in the context of advancing technology. *Journal of Law and the Biosciences, 7*(1), p. lsz016; Joly, Y., Feze, I.N. and Simard, J., 2013. Genetic discrimination and life insurance: a systematic review of the evidence. *BMC Medicine, 11*(1), pp. 1–15; Areheart, B.A. and Roberts, J.L., 2018. Gina, big data, and the future of employee privacy. *Yale LJ, 128*, p. 710.

95 Areheart, B.A. and Roberts, J.L., 2018. Gina, big data, and the future of employee privacy. *Yale LJ, 128*, p.710.

96 Future Advocacy., 2018. *Ethical, Social, and Political Challenges of Artificial Intelligence in Health*. A report with The Wellcome Trust. April 11, 2018. https://futureadvocacy.com/publications/ethical-social-and-political-challenges-of-artificial-intelligence-in-health/

97 West, S.M., Whittaker, M. and Crawford, K., 2019. Discriminating systems. *AI Now.*

98 Snow, J., 2018. 'We're in a diversity crisis': cofounder of Black in AI on what's poisoning algorithms in our lives. *MIT Technology Review*, February 14, 2018, https://www.technologyreview.com/s/610192/were-in-a-diversity-crisis-black-in-ais-founder-on-whats-poisoning-the-algorithms-in-our/

99 Marks, M., 2019. Tech companies are using AI to mine our digital traces. *STAT*, September 17, 2019 https://www.statnews.com/2019/09/17/digital-traces-tech-companies-artificial-intelligence/

100 Edwards, P.N., 2018. We have been assimilated: some principles for thinking about algorithmic systems," in *Living with Monsters? Social Implications of Algorithmic Phenomena, Hybrid Agency, and the Performativity of Technology*, Proceedings of the IFIP WG 8.2 Working Conference on the Interaction of Information Systems and the Organization, IS&O 2018, San Francisco, CA, USA, December 11–12, 2018, Ulrike Schultze, Margunn Aanestad, Magnus Mähring, Carsten Østerlund, Kai Riemer (eds.). Cham, Switzerland: Springer International Publishing.

101 Cho, G., Yim, J., Choi, Y., Ko, J., and Lee, S.H., 2019, April. Review of machine learning algorithms for diagnosing mental illness. *Psychiatry Investigation, 16*(4), pp. 262–269; Marks, M., 2019. Artificial intelligence based suicide prediction. *Yale Journal of Law and Technology, 21*, pp. 98–116; Chancellor, S., Birnbaum, M.L., Caine, E.D., Silenzio, V.M. and De Choudhury, M., 2019, January. A taxonomy of ethical tensions in inferring mental health states from social media. In *Proceedings of the Conference on Fairness, Accountability, and Transparency*, pp. 79–88.

102 Geis, J.R., Brady, A.P., Wu, C.C., Spencer, J., Ranschaert, E., Jaremko, J.L., Langer, S.G., Kitts, A.B., Birch, J., Shields, W.F. and van den Hoven van Genderen, R., 2019. Ethics of artificial intelligence in radiology: summary of the joint European and North American multisociety statement. *Canadian Association of Radiologists Journal, 70*(4), pp. 329–334.

103 Veinot, T.C., Mitchell, H. and Ancker, J.S., 2018. Good intentions are not enough: how informatics interventions can worsen inequality. *Journal of the American Medical Informatics Association, 25*(8), pp. 1080–1088; Kaziunas, E., Klinkman, M.S. and Ackerman, M.S., 2019. Precarious interventions: Designing for ecologies of care. *Proceedings of the ACM on Human-Computer Interaction, 3*(CSCW), pp. 1–27.

3 Organizational Change and Digital Maturity

How and why organizations change has been a central question for academics and practitioners alike across disciplines and sectors, including healthcare.[1] A longitudinal study of more than 1,000 organizations in 15 industries over a 36-year period showed that change is constant and often disruptive.[2] In both the Forbes 100 and the Standard and Poor's 500 lists, before the 1990s, most organizations such as DuPont, General Electric (GE), Johnson and Johnson and Procter & Gamble exhibited high productivity and earnings. As the study shows, during those years, vertical integration and other supply-driven forms of organizing, including a high ownership of assets across the supply chain, were key approaches to managing change. However, since the 1990s, market deregulation, technological advances and demand from different ecosystem actors including buyers, sellers, investors and customers generated a rate of change that outpaced the way organizations changed internally. Although some of these companies still exist today, most have either succumbed to market forces as in the case of Kodak, while others have had to diversify and split their multinational operations as in the case of GE. The key point made in this longitudinal study is that organizations must abandon the assumption of continuity that was so prevalent in the 20th century; instead they must understand and mitigate "cultural lock-in".[3] "Cultural lock-in results from the gradual stiffening of the invisible architecture of the corporation and the ossification of its decision-making abilities, control systems and mental models. It dampens a company's ability to innovate or to shed operations with a less-exciting future. Moreover, it signals the corporation's inexorable decline into inferior performance".[4] As others have noted, "over time (and even concurrently) organizations need evolution and revolution. When they have been limited exclusively to the restrictive precepts of social engineering, they have been handicapped and largely unsuccessful in unleashing authentic revolutionary change".[5]

Organizations like hospitals often engage in incremental improvements across their functional areas. For example, a hospital may plan the implementation of virtual clinics. The management team or the executive board of a hospital will have authority and control over the changes being proposed. At the same time, such proposed changes will be scrutinized by the external partners of the hospital and the broader market in which it operates. External partners such as digital service providers or medical device manufacturers will advise the choice of technologies to be implemented at the hospital, and will help define support and service level agreements, including pricing, as well as determine a timed implementation and rollout. Such incremental improvements will often be disrupted by market competition by startups who may enter the market with new technological innovations. Such change is disruptive because it is unanticipated both in its intention and time of occurrence. As a consequence of such market disruption,

DOI: 10.4324/9781032619569-4

healthcare service providers may engage in more revolutionary or transformative changes within their organization in order to respond and be able to compete. Patient demands, as in the case for more personalized services, may also disrupt incumbents, forcing them to implement changes that were not originally planned.[6]

This chapter discusses how healthcare organizations can lead change toward achieving higher value for patients. Value is discussed in relation to the healthcare delivery cycle, exploring how different ecosystem actors get involved in this cycle's distinct processes, going beyond healthcare service providers, to also examine the role of medical device manufacturers, diagnostic centers, biotech and pharmaceutical companies and digital service integrators, among others. Following this discussion, the focus shifts to how each of these ecosystem actors can develop unique value propositions by leveraging digital technology to achieve not only operational effectiveness at lower costs than competitors but also greater value for patients by delivering a better user experience).[7] The chapter outlines different levels of digital maturity, offering a blueprint by which healthcare organizations can identify where they stand and how they can begin to digitally transform themselves. The chapter concludes by discussing how new startups can use the assessment blueprint to craft comprehensive plans for becoming a digital-first organization.

3.1   The Healthcare Delivery Cycle: Co-Creating Value for Patients

Leading organizational change in healthcare starts with a process identification and analysis of the healthcare delivery cycle for each medical condition. By mapping the healthcare delivery cycle for each medical condition, organizations can achieve higher value for patients. Value is measured for the patient in relation to activities that help the prevention, early detection, right diagnosis and treatment for the patient, fewer complications and fewer errors in treatment, faster and more complete recovery, less disability and greater functionality with less need for long-term care. More healthy patients require fewer tests and fewer treatments and have fewer demands, thus lowering the overall costs of healthcare delivery.

Although each medical condition will include unique processes and activities, there are some broad process categories that can help structure a generic healthcare delivery cycle map as shown in Figure 3.1.

The healthcare delivery cycle involves five processes, namely, preventing, diagnosing, preparing, treating and recovering.[8] Each of these processes can be broken down into a set of activities that will vary depending on the medical condition. In addition, there are three sub-processes that cut across the five processes, namely, informing and engaging, measuring and accessing. These three sub-processes can be summarized in the following questions: (1) informing and engaging – what do patients need to be educated about? (2) measuring – what measures need to be collected about the patient's medical condition? and (3) accessing – where do care activities take place? These three cross-cutting sub-processes pervade all the main processes, that is, there is informing and engaging, measuring and accessing involved in preventing, diagnosing, preparing, treating and recovering. These sub-processes bind the healthcare delivery cycle together and are very much enabled by digital technology. They can help integrate the healthcare delivery cycle and digitally transform organizations to achieve higher patient value.

The healthcare delivery cycle begins with *preventing*, which includes a number of activities such as tracking a patient's biomarkers, assessing risk and taking steps to

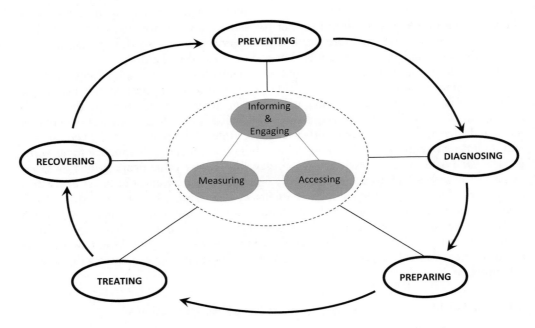

Figure 3.1 The Healthcare Delivery Cycle.

prevent or reduce the seriousness of illness or injury. Patients are increasingly becoming more *informed and engaged* about their health and wellness, using smart devices and wearables to track and *measure* their vital signals, including glucose levels, breathlessness and heart rates[9] and even *accessing* consultations about their genetic and genomic predisposition to diseases.[10] Healthcare providers are also becoming more engaged in the monitoring process, especially in relation to chronic conditions. For example, the Bristol Clinical Commissioning Group in the English NHS previously commissioned Safe Patient Systems to implement their Safe Mobile Care system[11] to monitor patients with chronic obstructive pulmonary disease (COPD) through their mobile phones. Vital signals such as blood pressure and weight were recorded, measured and communicated via the app, and the patients could also record their well-being (e.g., breathlessness). All patients participating in the project reported feeling empowered to manage their condition. There was 40 percent less nurse phone contact, 18 percent fewer nurse visits, 26 percent reduction in overall contact, 83 percent reduction in calls to GP and 57 percent reduction in visits to GP, alongside significant reduction of unplanned COPD admissions. Thus, with the help of smart devices and mobile apps, patients can participate in the monitoring of their own medical condition remotely. Occasionally, physical visits to a primary care or specialized doctor (in the case of specialized conditions) need to take place, exams taken, prescriptions provided and drugs administered. As the example from the Bristol Clinical Commissioning Group shows, in this process, it is not just the care providers that get involved, but also digital service providers such as Safe Patient Systems. Indeed, other ecosystem actors such as machine learning experts, bio-data banks and omics analysis specialists can enable healthcare providers to capture, combine and analyze multiple types of data that provide personalized simulations to predict the likely progression of chronic diseases in the future health of the patient.[12]

The next process is ***diagnosing,*** and it includes a number of activities such as physical examinations, tests and analysis of the patient's medical history potentially from multiple specialists. The accuracy of the diagnosis will significantly impact the value of care delivered in subsequent processes. Traditionally, diagnosing has been performed by large care provider centers such as hospitals, as well as by diagnostic centers, including medical imaging centers and biomedical labs. Patients are most usually *informed and engaged* about the results of these examinations by their doctors, who also communicate the final diagnosis to the patients. *Accessing* such examinations requires physical visits, and *measuring* the results is dependent on the availability of imaging specialists including radiologists, who then communicate results to the patients' doctors. Recent developments in the areas of chemical and biochemical sensors, lab-on-a-chip systems, Internet of Things (IoT) technology and wearable electronics have enabled new approaches for mobile and wearable point of care diagnostic devices (POCD). A mobile or wearable POCD device is a standalone mobile system such as a smartphone which can read measurement signals of target patients from samples collected in a sensing platform and send detection results to care providers or diagnostic centers via wireless communication. Sensitive and reliable POCD have been commercialized for remote diagnostics including detection of anaemia, prostate cancer, HIV and syphilis, among others.[13] With the advent of genomic technologies like next-generation sequencing, combined with an increased interest in precision medicine, there have been significant developments in POCD tests involving genomic methods. In particular, analysis of circulating tumor cells and cell-free DNA is becoming increasingly popular for POCD devices.[14]

In addition to POCD that expand the ways by which the sub-processes of informing and engaging, accessing and measuring can be performed, diagnosing is being augmented via artificial intelligence (AI) technologies. Radiologists and histopathologists around the world are faced with an ever-increasing volume of imaging data. AI technologies are being deployed to augment the diagnosing process by processing routine cases, thus minimizing the work of the human specialists. AI technologies can highlight high-risk cases and alert radiologists and histopathologists to examine these cases in more depth. For example, Moorfields Eye Hospital in London has partnered with DeepMind[15] to use an AI-augmented optical coherence tomography (OCT) to diagnose retinal diseases. Other healthcare providers lacking retina specialists can enter into a partnership with Moorfields Eye Hospital to outsource their diagnosing process. This expands the level of access to such diagnosing for individual patients, even in remote locations.

Preparing is placed in between diagnosing and treating, as it comes after a doctor has communicated available treatment plans for the patient's medical condition and before a treatment is chosen and performed. Careful preparation before treatment can significantly improve health outcomes. For example, in the case of severe knee osteoarthritis and depending on the surgical options (e.g., minimally invasive or open knee for a knee replacement) the patient will need to have blood tests performed, pre-op physical exams and cardiac and pulmonary evaluations. *Measuring* the outcomes of these preparatory exams will impact which treatment option(s) become viable, especially in relation to the patient's overall physical condition and other comorbidities. Other medical conditions such as breast cancer will require different preparations such as testing for postmenopausal hormonal imbalance or a medical history in the family for Hodgin's disease. In preparing patients for intervention, they need to be *informed and engaged* about their options, set expectations and also, in some cases, be referred to psychological counseling. For example, breast cancer will often necessitate complete removal of the breast (mastectomy) to avoid complications including metastasis, but this will then require subsequent oncoplastic surgery for breast reconstruction. The life-threatening, aesthetic and cost-related considerations often cause mental health issues in patients.[16] *Accessing* all these preparatory exams and consultations has previously been bound to physical visits. However, more recently, the use of telehealth and virtual psychiatry consultations for women with breast cancer has been found to have positive effects on treatment-related psychological conditions.[17] This is also true for other types of medical conditions.

Following the preparing process, **treating** involves activities for reversing or mitigating a medical condition by offering drug therapy, surgery, chemotherapy or other such treatments to patients. Treatments are usually *accessed* physically in an operating theater, an oncology center and pharmacies in the case of simple drug therapies. *Measurements* such as blood loss during surgery, complications or drug side effects are taken to assess the patient's response to the treatment. Patients are *informed and engaged* about the effects of their treatment, as well as how to manage their expectations for recovery. The treating process will involve a number of specialists (e.g., in breast cancer these could be gynecologists, oncologists and general surgeons), but also pharmaceutical, biotech and prosthetic companies. Indeed, in the case of experimental treatments, patients may be given the option to participate in early clinical trials of new drugs. Biotech companies have developed AI technologies to discover new targets, design new drugs and predict the outcomes of clinical trials cutting down the time and cost to bring new life-saving drugs to market.[18] Such technologies often utilize semantic and natural language processing approaches to combine clinical trial data from past drug discovery processes with pharmacogenomic data, electronic patient records and the scientific literature, allowing for further annotations of clinical candidates with molecular targets.[19] This means that patients and their treating doctors have access to better, more in-depth measurements to allow them to make more informed decisions. Indeed, AI technologies are also used to design more dynamic treatment regimes such as managing the rates of reintubation and regulating physiological stability in intensive care units.[20] Finally, augmented and virtual reality technologies are used to enhance surgical training[21] and improve understanding of different treatment options.[22]

Recovering follows any treatment that has been provided to the patient. It starts from the moment the patient leaves the surgery room or stops chemotherapy sessions and completes a drug therapy and could involve rehabilitation, physical therapy and daily living support. Managing recovery well can have a significant impact on health outcomes, while reducing re-hospitalization due to complications. *Informing and engaging* patients on their rehabilitation programs and setting expectations on their longitudinal care plans is an important subprocess. Also, *measuring* data post-treatment such as symptoms and function, pain and the ability to return to normal routines is paramount. *Accessing* such services for recovery can happen both at a rehabilitation facility or even at a care center, but also at home. Indeed, for more than a decade or so, augmented reality technologies have been used to support the rehabilitation programs of patients with various medical conditions, including those who previously suffered a stroke[23] or those suffering from neurological diseases.[24]

Recovering feeds into a new cycle of prevention by continuing to monitor the patient's overall health and well-being. The key objective is to reduce the possibility of further disease acceleration and subsequent treatment. Certainly, a patient may suffer from multiple comorbidities, and thus, the healthcare delivery cycle is iterative and constant, requiring existing and new ecosystem actors to get involved in the management of the medical condition. Ongoing monitoring and diagnosing (e.g., annual mammograms to detect breast cancer) is essential for prevention of disease and for achieving higher value for patients.

Leading organizational change in healthcare requires an in-depth analysis of the healthcare delivery cycle to understand where improvements can be made, which eco-system actors to engage and how to measure value and at what costs. At the very core of the healthcare delivery cycle lies patient data that provides rich insights into the complex nature of health and disease. A patient's data needs to be regarded as a living resource, with new data, be they from a sensor, results of a lab test or genomic analysis using machine learning, being combined with old data, while providing an end-to-end, seamless experience to patients. To achieve such end-to-end, seamless experience, organizations need to become digitally mature, deploying a number of different tech-nologies like the ones discussed above across the healthcare delivery cycle.

3.2   Achieving Digital Maturity in Healthcare Organizations

Leadership decisions to achieve digital maturity will lead to changes in strategy, as well as the human and technological capabilities needed to perform different activities within the healthcare delivery cycle.

As defined in Chapter 1, **digital maturity** is the *measure of an organization's capabilities to create and capture value by leveraging digital technologies.* Such capabilities need to be developed with appropriate governance rules that will enable value creation and capture. Digital maturity can be measured across the three dimensions of strategy, human capabilities and technology capabilities as deployed in the five processes of the healthcare delivery cycle.

Decisions on changing the three dimensions of digital maturity will vary in their complexity and impact depending on who is making them, from entrepreneurs seeking solution partners to their biotechnology innovations, to clinical leads in different sec-ondary care departments within hospitals making decisions on which workflow system to select, to business unit leaders within medical device manufacturer divisions choosing which third parties to partner with, and to chief executives in private and national insurance organizations making decisions on which products and services to discontinue and launch. These and other such leadership decisions will be faced with unique risks and opportunities and will involve input from various individuals, teams and depart-ments within relevant organizations.

Leadership decisions are made by leaders at the very top of the organization who define the "mental structures" that activate the rest of the organization's skills and competencies, but also their expectations and obligations.[25] These mental structures form the identity – "who we are", "what we believe and want" and "how we prefer to be seen by the outside world" as an organization.[26] In turn, this identity helps to define the vision of the orga-nization in the form of its core value proposition. For example, Bill Gates' vision of Microsoft reflected a core value proposition to build a product (i.e., software) ecosystem that would serve a growing number of business users (primarily enterprise organizations) and their heterogeneous needs, while also enabling third-party developers to complement that ecosystem with additional products and services.[27] In contrast, Steve Jobs' vision of Apple reflected a core value proposition of building, first a product (i.e., hardware devices) and then a platform ecosystem (i.e., its iOS and App Store) to provide a seamless ex-perience for end-users.[28]

The questions of "who we are", "what we believe and want" and "how we prefer to be seen by the outside world" as an organization reflect an understanding of the internal resources and capabilities of the organization and the services and products it can offer. For example, the Mayo Clinic, a large healthcare service organization operating across three campuses, 70 hospitals and several medical colleges, places the needs of the patients first.[29] This strategic vision is "driven into the operations, into the policy, into the decision making, into the allocation of resources, and ultimately into the culture of the organization", as Dr. Glenn S. Forbes, CEO of Mayo Clinic in Rochester explained.[30] The Mayo Clinic Model of Care incorporates specific principles of how patient care should be delivered, evaluated and improved, and how staff should be trained and nurtured to grow into professional leaders, as well as how technology should be used to augment such growth. Indeed, the value proposition of a healthcare organization cuts across the five processes of the healthcare delivery cycle.

Key to organizational change is the ability to change the individual knowledge, attitudes and behavior of people in organizations all of which impact job motivation and specific task performance that are relevant to organizational functioning and effectiveness.[31] It is not possible for organizations to change in meaningful ways unless people change. Organizations change people in many ways including socialization processes, training and supervision.[32] At the same time, changing people changes organizations. In other words, there is a reciprocal relationship between the change that individuals experience in the workplace with the change that organizations undergo over time. The degree to which individuals change has been found to vary according to their personality traits, including their extrinsic and intrinsic motivations to change.[33] For example, individuals find it easier to change their task-specific behavior than their norm-regulated behavior that is embedded in social relationships and organizational values.[34] Indeed, if the change program fundamentally questions individuals' perceptions of their identity or even their organization's identity, it is met with significant resistance and may take considerable time to be implemented.[35]

One study found that perceived identity reinforcements and deteriorations in change programs had a significant impact in the assimilation of electronic health records (EHR) in physician practices.[36] In particular, the study found that when change was consistent with referent others and enhanced physicians' standing within their group, they openly embraced EHR, whereas when change was perceived as intrusive to their identity, physicians took action to preserve their identity from threats. This explains why some organizations take less time to implement change, in particular technological change: if technological innovation and transformation embed the core identity traits of the organization, and if such transformation is not challenging to individuals' own identities, individuals find it easier to adopt new technologies.

Evidently,[37] organizations will exhibit different levels of digital maturity, and this will impact their readiness for digital transformation. Table 3.1 provides a summary of an organization's digital maturity, from low to high, across the five processes of the healthcare delivery cycle and according to the three dimensions of strategy, human capabilities and technology capabilities. The sections that follow provide more details with examples to help organizations understand their digital maturity.

Arguably, a healthcare organization can exhibit high digital maturity in one process (e.g., diagnosing) and one dimension (e.g., technology capabilities) while exhibiting medium or even low digital maturity in other processes and dimensions. Identifying where in the digital maturity spectrum a healthcare organization stands will have

Table 3.1 Levels of Digital Maturity in Healthcare Organizations: An Assessment Blueprint

Low Digital Maturity	*Medium Digital Maturity*	*High Digital Maturity*
Strategy	**Strategy**	**Strategy**
• Unclear strategy across the healthcare delivery cycle	• Basic strategy for digitally supporting the healthcare delivery cycle	• Comprehensive and well-defined strategy for digitally supporting the healthcare delivery cycle
• No clear goals or ecosystem-wide coordination	• Limited participation in digital projects with third-party partners, but these projects are not integrated with other systems in the organization	• Participation in ecosystems or orchestration of own ecosystem with clearly defined value propositions
• No understanding of how the data collected across the healthcare delivery cycle can generate important insights that can feed into new digital services	• Limited understanding of potentially new value creation streams from digital innovations and digital data	• Established data culture with clear strategic goals and governance rules to achieve high value creation and capture
Human Capabilities	**Human Capabilities**	**Human Capabilities**
• Staff members are not trained in the use of digital technology to support the healthcare delivery cycle	• Staff members have limited training in the use of digital technology to support the healthcare delivery cycle	• Staff members are highly trained and skilled in the use of digital technology to support the healthcare delivery cycle
• Internal standalone teams use conventional technology or outsource their needs to third parties	• There is a dedicated digital unit that is responsible for digitally supporting parts of the healthcare delivery cycle	• Every functional area has a digital unit with a range of digital capabilities including software development and data analytics
• There is no dedicated digital leader nor a digital unit for augmenting the healthcare delivery cycle	• No capabilities for in-house software development and data analytics	• Both staff and patients are supported in a flexible, continuous and responsive way
• Data are not captured systematically by staff neither integrated into technology systems such as electronic patient records.	• Some data insights are missed	**Technology Capabilities**
Technology Capabilities	**Technology Capabilities**	• Access to a full range of digital technology to support the healthcare delivery cycle
• No access to digital technology such as AI, smart devices, intelligent sensors and robotic systems to support the healthcare delivery cycle	• Access to limited digital technology to support the healthcare delivery cycle	• Intelligent sensors are deployed in healthcare organizations and even in patient homes with patients' informed consent to capture data
• No integration with external partners' digital technologies and applications	• Parts of the technology infrastructure are hosted on the cloud and can support digital applications for limited pilots with limited data analytics capabilities	• Machine learning models are deployed across the healthcare delivery cycle and data are integrated across functional areas to enable cross-disciplinary insights
• Legacy technology infrastructure is situated in organizational premises with often siloed systems and data centers	• The technology infrastructure is not governed or architected for scale, reliability and security	• The technology infrastructure is scalable, reliable and secure and provides integration across the healthcare delivery cycle

implications for its ability to implement important changes to improve the healthcare delivery cycle.

3.2.1 Healthcare Organizations with Low Digital Maturity

3.2.1.1 Preventing

Healthcare organizations with low digital maturity do not have a clear strategy in place for digitally monitoring patients' health and wellness and preventing disease. Organizations such as national and regional hospitals and national payers will depend on aggregated, periodic, population health-level data, often provided by third parties such as the World Health Organization[38] or independent analysts,[39] to monitor patients. In such cases, there are no clear goals or ecosystem-wide coordination efforts to improve patient monitoring.

These organizations do not have the human capabilities to support the monitoring of patients' health and wellness. Most staff members are not trained in the use of digital technology and patients often report their symptoms to these organizations through physical visits. This is typical of public sector primary care centers around the world, especially those suffering from low human resources, lack of funding and IT support.[40] In these cases, data is not captured systematically by staff, neither is it integrated into technology systems such as electronic patient records. Exactly because of the lack of human resources and the amount of work that healthcare professionals are already subjected to, there is no time nor the funding to assign a dedicated digital leader or to develop a digital unit that would be responsible for the digital monitoring of patients' health and wellness for preventing disease.

Healthcare organizations with low digital maturity do not have access to digital technology such as smart wearable devices and intelligent sensors to support the monitoring of patients' health and wellness, whether remotely or in organizational premises. There is often a legacy technology infrastructure situated in organizational premises that does not have capabilities for integrating third-party apps for patient monitoring and prevention. Even in cases where such integration is intended, the process is resource-intensive and subject to various technical and organizational challenges. For example, research into the monitoring of elderly patients in their homes through "ambient assisted living" technologies has pointed at the heterogeneity of devices and standards involved that often challenge the integration of several subsystems within the home.[41] Patients are often confronted with a non-homogeneous interface and non-seamless use of these "ambient assisted living" technologies. In consequence, few such technologies are scaled up beyond their initial proof-of-concept studies.[42] Unless organizations partner with other ecosystem partners for fully integrated solutions, there is poor coordination and efficiency in the preventing process that often leads to poor outcomes in preventing disease.

3.2.1.2 Diagnosing

As with the previous process, healthcare organizations with low digital maturity do not have a strategy in place for augmenting diagnostic tests and exams with digital technologies. There is often a lack of understanding of how the diagnosing process can generate important data that can feed into new digital services. A recent report by KPMG shows that despite a rising demand for more diagnostic tests in "most of the world's largest healthcare economies, many diagnostics companies face a continuing struggle against commoditization", because public and private payers are always seeking "regular price cuts, with diagnostics too often viewed as a relatively easy source of additional savings".[43] Most importantly, such cuts means that the huge opportunities offered by digital technologies in augmenting diagnostic tests and exams are missed and so are the data insights that can potentially be generated.

These organizations have staff members who are not trained in the use of digital technology for augmenting diagnostic tests and exams. Rather, their staff are organized in standalone diagnostic teams (e.g., pathology, radiology) that provide diagnostic tests with conventional technology. In cases where healthcare organizations do not even have such human capabilities (e.g., lacking MRI radiologists and medical devices), they outsource their diagnostic needs to external diagnostic centers. In fact, purchasing and running diagnostic technology such as MRI and CT scans is very expensive for some resource-constrained healthcare organizations that often resort to outsourcing imaging services from third parties.[44]

Healthcare organizations with low digital maturity do not have access to digital technology for augmenting diagnostic tests and exams. Those that do own and operate diagnostic technology rely on medical device manufacturers for technical support, but often such technology is not integrated into other technologies in the organization such as electronic patient records. This may result in data not being collected, processed and analyzed for cross-disciplinary insights into different medical conditions, but more critically, it can also lead to diagnostic errors.[45] Although there are many available standards for diagnostic technologies, including interfaces that can enable seamless integration between information systems, there are still healthcare organizations whose technology infrastructure for supporting diagnostic tests is separate from other technologies in the organization. This can result in a lack of coordination and efficiency in the diagnostic process and can lead to poor diagnostic outcomes.

3.2.1.3 *Preparing*

The preparing process is most often supported by specialized teams of professionals that are often situated outside focal healthcare organizations and who are assigned the task to prepare patients for their upcoming treatment work. For example, there is a growing body of research on the preparation or "prehabilitation" of newly diagnosed cancer patients and how that affects their health prior to starting acute treatments.[46] This research reports on the role of psychologists, nutritionists and fitness professionals in "optimizing" patient outcomes by improving overall fitness levels, including muscle function, oxygen saturation, breathing, range of motion and stress coping, among others. Because these "prehabilitation" interventions take place outside the organizations offering the actual treatment, there is little strategic interest to invest in digital technology for digitally preparing patients for different treatment options. This process is controlled exclusively by third parties.

Accordingly, organizational staff members are not trained in the use of digital technology for preparing patients for different treatment options. Patients are referred to specialized staff external to the organization. There are no digital skills and capabilities for supporting virtual consultations and counseling in preparing patients for treatment. There is really no interest from top management to develop such teams and capabilities because of the perception that no added value can be gained from doing so.

By extension, healthcare organizations with a low digital maturity have no access to such digital technology as virtual and augmented reality technologies, as well as AI-enabled chatbots or robots to assist in the preparing process. The technology infrastructure of the organization does not support any such technologies. This can result in a lack of support and guidance for patients and can potentially lead to poor health outcomes.

3.2.1.4 *Treating*

Healthcare organizations may be best in class in offering different treatment options to patients, from surgery, chemotherapy or other types of treatments, but they may suffer from a low digital maturity. Such organizations do not have a clear strategy in place for augmenting treatment options with digital technology as in the example of robotic surgery. Exactly because of an unclear strategy, such organizations also lack an understanding of how the treating process can generate important data that can feed into new digital services. For example, a recent study has reported how missing data on hospital-based hand surgery can generate poor analyses of postoperative morbidity and thus fail to predict major complications.[47]

Similar to the rest of the discussion on healthcare organizations with low digital maturity, such organizations have staff members who are not trained in the use of digital technology for augmenting treatment options. There may be internal standalone teams that provide treatment with conventional technology. In cases where healthcare organizations do not even have such human capabilities, they outsource their treatment needs to external partners and that is when data insights from the treating process may be completely lost, as one study of patient referrals for cancer treatment in Brazil has recently shown.[48]

Organizations with low digital maturity do not have access to digital technology for augmenting treatment options. They may also suffer from no integration with external partners' systems, thus impacting patient flow.[49] Because of the lack of interoperability with other technologies in the organization and with partners' systems, data is not collected, processed and analyzed for cross-disciplinary insights into the treatment of different medical conditions, including postoperative complications. This can result in a lack of coordination and efficiency in the treatment process and can lead to poor treatment outcomes and even high patient mortality. One study found that in organizations where there was no surveillance monitoring of patients undergoing sedative/analgesic treatment in the general care setting experienced 19.73 deaths per 100,000 at risk patients, as opposed to organizations that used surveillance monitoring of such treatments.[50]

3.2.1.5 *Recovering*

Finally, healthcare organizations with low digital maturity have no clear strategy for providing rehabilitation and recovery for patients. As in the case of the preparing process, the recovering process is most often exclusively controlled by third parties who have the expertise and capabilities to rehabilitate patients after the treatment. As such, organizations have no strategic interest to invest in digital technology for digital recovering.

By extension, organizations have no staff members who are trained in the use of digital technology for providing rehabilitation and recovery for patients. There are no digital skills and capabilities for supporting digital recovering services. Patients are referred to specialized staff external to the organization. Once again, this means that there are no data insights gained from this process, even if data is shared by third parties through the patient.

A recent review of research on patients that developed postoperative atrial fibrillation after cardiac surgery found that implanted devices allowing the continual monitoring of patients at risk of this complication could "pickup much more brief paroxysmal episodes than intermittent sampling" through physical monitoring.[51] However, such opportunities are missed in healthcare organizations with low digital maturity that do not have access to such digital technologies for monitoring rehabilitation and recovery for patients. The technology infrastructure does not support digital technologies for digital recovering services both within organizational premises and across partners. This can result in a lack of support and guidance for patients during this critical phase of their healthcare journey and can lead to poor recovery outcomes.

3.2.2   Healthcare Organizations with Medium Digital Maturity

3.2.2.1   Preventing

Healthcare organizations with a medium level of digital maturity have a basic strategy in place for digitally monitoring patients' health and wellness and preventing disease. However, this strategy might not be comprehensive or well-defined. For example, organizations participate in digital projects that track patients' well-being and medical conditions, but these projects are not integrated with other systems. The Bristol NHS Trust project discussed earlier came to an end in 2017 and although it reported positive outcomes for patients in the five years of its operation, it was discontinued after the funding ended. Safe Patient Systems was dissolved in 2019.[52]

Such projects as the one in Bristol may help organizations develop some human capabilities in the use of digital technology to support the monitoring of patients' health and wellness and preventing disease, but this training might be limited or short-lived and not systematized in organizational routines. There may be a dedicated digital unit that is responsible for the monitoring of patients, often placed within the IT department of the organization. This unit may also incorporate nursing or clinical leaders who are responsible for pilot projects. These healthcare professionals are trained to use the technology and deliver digital monitoring solutions, but the rest of the staff in the organization have no such training or understanding of the technology. In addition, the technology professionals in the digital unit do not have capabilities for in-house software development and data analytics. As a consequence, some insights are not captured from such projects.

Accordingly, organizations with medium digital maturity may have access to some digital technology to support the monitoring of patients' health and wellness for preventing disease, but this technology is limited and not comprehensive. Parts of the technology infrastructure are hosted on the cloud and can support telehealth and potentially even IoT applications for limited pilots.[53] However, this technology infrastructure is not governed or architected for scale, reliability and security across the organization. This can lead to a lack of consistency and effectiveness in the preventing process and can result in suboptimal outcomes in preventing disease.

3.2.2.2   Diagnosing

Organizations have a basic strategy in place for augmenting diagnostic tests and exams with digital technologies, but this strategy might not be comprehensive or well-defined. There are partnerships in place with diagnostic centers and medical device manufacturers for ad hoc support of digital diagnostics through AI workflow systems, but there is limited strategic positioning in identifying new value creation streams from digital innovations. As discussed earlier, profit margins have dropped in the diagnostics market which are impairing the ability of diagnostic and medical device manufacturers to innovate.[54] Chapter 2 has already discussed the problem of overprescribing tests and the rising costs to healthcare services. The implication is that even organizations with medium digital maturity are keen to curb excessive diagnosing. As a consequence, there have been a lot of acquisitions and mergers in the diagnostics market by means of minimizing costs and achieving economies of scale.[55] This trend puts pressure on diagnostics firms to build stronger relationships with other ecosystem actors including payers, healthcare providers, doctors and even patients to develop strategies for digital solutions that will be more efficient, both in terms of cost and health outcomes.

At the same time, as the diagnosing process is outsourced to specialized diagnostic centers, healthcare organizations are struggling to train new, internal diagnostics staff. The Royal College of Radiologists (RCR) in the UK has reported in 2021 that the NHS needs nearly 2,000 more radiologists.[56] The RCR 2021 Census reports that "without more consultants in training, investment in new models of care and better staff retention and recruitment, by 2025 the UK's radiologist shortfall will hit 44% (3,613 consultants short of real terms demand)".[57] Similar numbers are reported across the world.[58] What this means is that even in the case of organizations with medium digital maturity, although there may be some staff members who have some training in the use of digital technology for augmenting diagnostic tests and exams, these staff members are not able to cover the diagnostic needs of their organization. Once again, cost considerations together with a very low number of diagnostic staff in training and in residency positions push organizations to outsource their diagnostic needs to large diagnostic centers.

Having said this, organizations with medium digital maturity have dedicated digital training programs with which to augment their diagnostic staff to be able to coordinate with external partners. For example, Brigham & Women's Hospital in the USA designed a data science pathway for the resident radiologists that combines "formal instruction and practical problem-solving collaborations with data scientists, exposing residents to all aspects of AI-ML application development, including data curation, model design, quality control, and clinical testing".[59] Although help and support from external partners is still required, such training programs help to build some initial human capabilities for augmenting diagnostic tests and exams with digital technology.

Following from the above discussion, organizations with medium digital maturity have some access to digital technology for augmenting diagnostic tests and exams, but this technology might be limited and not comprehensive. A limited number of machine learning models are used with diagnostic data for a small number of medical conditions or for supporting the training of diagnostic staff as in the case of Brigham & Women's Hospital. These department or unit-based models are hosted on the cloud and support limited integrations with AI workflow systems from third parties. However, this infrastructure is not governed or architected for scale, reliability and security. For example, organizations may not have clear governance rules for diagnostic data such as medical images, and there may be issues of securing the privacy of sensitive patient data. This can lead to a lack of consistency and effectiveness in the diagnostic process and can result in suboptimal diagnostic outcomes.

3.2.2.3 *Preparing*

Organizations have a basic strategy in place for digitally preparing patients for different treatment options, but this strategy might not be comprehensive or well-defined. There are partnerships in place with external patient-facing platforms, but there is limited strategic positioning in identifying new value creation streams from digital innovations. For example, organizations such as the ALS Hope Foundation, the Lupus Foundation of Northern California, King's College London, the National Institute of Mental Health and many more[60] have partnered with PatientsLikeMe (recently acquired by UnitedHealth Group[61]) to receive aggregated data that they can use to improve their research and development on preparing their patients. Platforms like PatientsLikeMe benefit from people providing their own personal data with their informed consent to be used to support other patients living with chronic conditions. Such partnerships with external patient-facing platforms are definitely better than nothing, but they are often not integrated with other strategic objectives across the organization.

Exactly because aggregated data from external partners often do not feed into other functional areas and information systems such as electronic patient records, the data lacks confounding interactions between the progression of disease on a particular patient and the interventions that are needed to manage that disease. Thus, patients are prepared on the basis of patterns found in a patient population, patterns that may miss specific guidance for individual patients. Staff in organizations with medium digital maturity may have some training in the use of digital technology for preparing patients for different treatment options. However, their role and capabilities is reduced to coordinating with external platforms while lacking close engagement with data that would provide intelligence and specificity for preparing individual patients.

Accordingly, organizations with medium digital maturity have limited access to digital technology for preparing patients for different treatment options. Some applications and digital services are not supported, neither is data securely stored. The infrastructure is not governed or architected for scale, reliability and security. This can lead to a lack of consistency in the support and guidance provided to patients and can result in sub-optimal health outcomes.

3.2.2.4 *Treating*

Healthcare organizations with medium digital maturity have a basic strategy in place for augmenting treatment options with digital technology, even though this strategy may not integrate very well with other strategic objectives. For example, in recent years, many hospitals have started experimenting with the use of augmented and virtual reality technologies to assist different treatments. One study examined the use of virtual reality technologies "in adults with chronic pain, who have high disability and high fear of movement and reinjury".[62] The study used a double-blind, randomized, controlled trial to show that the technology helped participants reduce their fear of movement, minimize their pain intensity and pain interference from baseline measures. Although promising, such studies need to be protocolized, automated and scaled such that they become part of everyday routines. This requires strategic intent but also willingness from patients to participate. Exactly because hospitals often do not have the digital maturity to run such studies and to develop relevant technologies they partner with technology companies to realize this potential. Companies like XRHealth are beginning to create virtual reality clinics that help hospitals provide remote care to their patients throughout the USA, while partnering with major health insurance companies as well as national payers like Medicare.[63]

Following from the above example, organizations with medium digital maturity depend on external partners to offer the necessary training to staff members to learn to use of digital technology for augmenting treatment options. For example, XRHealth offers such training to clinicians to be able to monitor their patients' live virtual reality treatment sessions remotely, while also making adjustments in the process.[64] Similarly, FundamentalVR offers a virtual reality medical training platform that augments surgeons' capabilities in conducting different types of surgeries across urology, ophthalmology, orthopedics, spine and endovascular.[65] However, in both cases, hospitals would not have the capabilities to develop their own technology solutions, analyze data and support patients. These are capabilities offered by their external partners. Indeed, companies like XRHealth can directly manage individual patient's treatment plans via private insurance companies. Thus, healthcare organizations such as hospitals may lose access to the patient treatment experience altogether and with it valuable data.

Accordingly, healthcare organizations with medium digital maturity have some access to digital technology for augmenting treatment options, but this technology is most often hosted on an external partner's platform. Although there may be opportunities to integrate such platforms with the internal technology infrastructure, healthcare organizations depend on external partners' capabilities. The secured storing of data including data analysis and the management of the patient experience sits within the technology infrastructure of external partners. This can lead to a lack of consistency and effectiveness in the treatment process and can result in suboptimal treatment outcomes, especially in the case of patients with multiple comorbidities requiring treatment in other healthcare organizations than the external partners.

3.2.2.5 *Recovering*

Comprehensive recovering has been recognized as the most cost-effective intervention to ensure improved outcomes across different medical conditions. Such improvements include lower morbidity, decreased hospital admissions, increased physiological and psychological well-being and health span. However, as discussed earlier, recovering and rehabilitation is usually delivered in hospital outpatient departments, community centers and in some parts of the world as inpatient services. These center-based rehabilitation programmes, however, suffer from poor participation. For example, cardiac rehabilitation suffers from a lower than 20 percent participation in both the USA and Europe.[66] In response to such low numbers, national standard and professional bodies have called for the need of virtual technologies for home-based rehabilitation facilitated by healthcare professionals.[67] Companies like InMotion VR are offering solutions to augment the recovering process through home-based interventions.[68] Once again, such partnerships between healthcare organizations and technology vendors offer a basic strategy for augmenting rehabilitation and recovery for patients. Such arms-length partnerships may lack integration with other digital strategy initiatives within the organization.

Healthcare organizations with medium digital maturity have staff members who have some training in the use of digital technology for providing rehabilitation and recovery for patients. However, this training is usually offered by external partners and not integrated within the organization as part of other digital training. For example, MindMaze, a company offering virtual reality technologies for neuro-rehabilitation, is currently working with hospitals around the world to train clinicians and patients in the use of different applications across in-patient, post-acute and home-based care environments.[69] Recovering and rehabilitation protocols are developed in partnership with leading healthcare centers such as the John Hopkins and Mount Sinai hospitals in the USA. Healthcare organizations can begin to develop digital units and assign digital leaders across different departments through such external partnerships; however, this requires extensive training and recruitment that may take time to achieve.

Healthcare organizations with medium digital maturity have some access to digital technology for providing rehabilitation and recovery for patients, but this technology might be limited and not comprehensive. A limited number of applications are used for a small number of medical conditions or for supporting the training of staff. These department or unit-based applications are hosted on the cloud through external partners and support limited integrations with other technology systems within the organization, including those provided by third parties. This technology infrastructure is not governed or architected for scale, reliability and security. This can lead to a lack of consistency and effectiveness in the support provided to patients and can result in suboptimal recovery outcomes.

3.2.3 *Healthcare Organizations with High Digital Maturity*

Healthcare organizations with high digital maturity have comprehensive and well-defined strategies that allow them to effectively use technology to augment all five processes of the healthcare delivery cycle. Such organizations participate in ecosystems or even orchestrate their own ecosystem with clearly defined goals and business use cases. They also have a combination of human and technology capabilities with which to improve patient outcomes, reduce healthcare costs and raise the overall quality of care.

Examples of such healthcare organizations include the Cleveland Clinic[70] and the Mayo Clinic[71] in the USA, the Royal Marsden NHS Foundation Trust in the UK,[72] Ping An HealthKonnect and JD Health in China,[73] Seoul National University Bundang Hospital in South Korea,[74] the Karolinska University Hospital in Sweden,[75] and the Mulk e-hospital in the United Arab Emirates[76] among many more. These organizations have deployed such digital technologies as remote monitoring platforms that use wearable devices and smartphones to track patients' vital signs and activity levels across a variety of medical conditions; they have implemented AI-powered diagnostic tools that use machine learning algorithms to analyze radiologic images and to combine insights from electronic patient records; they have developed digital care planning systems that allow healthcare professionals to create individualized care plans for patients and share them with other specialists for collaboration and consultation; they have used robotic systems and minimally invasive surgical techniques to perform more precise and accurate treatments, leading to improved patient outcomes and faster recovery times; and they have deployed augmented and virtual reality technologies to provide follow-up care and rehabilitation for patients enabling an improved continuity of care and more efficient recovery for patients. These organizations are also exemplars in developing digital training programs that run across their departments and that are supported by digital leaders with strong capabilities and skills in deploying and using the aforementioned technologies.

3.2.3.1 *Preventing*

Organizations with high digital maturity have a comprehensive and well-defined strategy in place for digitally monitoring patients' health and wellness and preventing disease. These organizations participate in ecosystems or even orchestrate their own ecosystem with clearly defined goals and business use cases on patient monitoring. Partners in these ecosystems include medical device manufacturers that can provide healthcare organizations with advanced medical technologies such as wearable sensors and remote monitoring systems. Further, digital service providers can provide expertise and support in the development of algorithms and analytics systems that can support the analysis of data. These ecosystem partnerships are defined with clear strategic goals and governance rules in place to achieve high value creation and capture in the monitoring process. For example, by using wearable monitors and remote monitoring systems, they can track patients' vital signs and activity levels in real time, allowing them to quickly identify any changes in a patient's condition and take appropriate action. This can lead to early detection and intervention of potential health issues, reducing the need for more costly and invasive treatments down the line. Additionally, by using these technologies, healthcare providers can monitor patients with chronic conditions more effectively, preventing complications and hospitalization and in turn reducing healthcare costs.

Organizations have staff members who are highly trained and skilled in the use of digital technology to support the monitoring of patients' health and wellness for preventing disease. They have a team of trained healthcare professionals who are able to interpret and act on the data collected by the monitoring technology. They also have a team of data analysts who can use data analytics to gain insights into population health, identify trends and patterns and improve the overall quality of care. Additionally, they have a team of IT professionals who can manage and maintain the technology infrastructure and ensure that the systems are secure and compliant with relevant regulations. Patients are supported in a flexible, continuous and responsive way in monitoring their own health and wellness and preventing disease.

Organizations have access to a full range of digital technology to support the prevention process. For example, smart tracking systems and mobile apps are used by patients in their own personal, smart devices and these can communicate with patient facing applications controlled by healthcare organizations. Intelligent sensors are deployed in healthcare organizations such as hospitals and even in patient homes with patients' informed consent to capture monitoring data. Such monitoring feeds into the rest of the processes of the healthcare delivery cycle and is integrated in scalable, reliable and secure infrastructure. This infrastructure can provide a structured and coordinated approach to monitoring and can help ensure the best possible outcomes in preventing disease.

3.2.3.2 *Diagnosing*

Organizations have a comprehensive and well-defined strategy in place for augmenting diagnostic tests and exams with digital technologies across their ecosystem. For example, partners such as genomics and machine learning experts can provide healthcare organizations with advanced technologies and techniques that can support the analysis and interpretation of genetic data, which can help healthcare providers understand a patient's individual characteristics and needs. Further, biotech and device manufacturers provide POCD devices for remote diagnostic services. These ecosystem partnerships are defined with clear strategic goals and governance rules in place to achieve high value creation and capture in the diagnosing process. Overall, organizations with high digital maturity in diagnosing have a clear strategy with which to improve the accuracy and timeliness of diagnoses, facilitate collaboration and consultation among specialists and improve the patient experience, which leads to improved patient outcomes and reduction in healthcare costs.

Organizations have staff members who are highly trained and skilled in the use of digital technology for augmenting diagnostic tests and exams. Staff such as radiologists and microbiologists work closely with data scientists to augment the analysis of their tests and exams and produce intelligent insights in the diagnosing process. There are dedicated leaders in each diagnostic area and even skilled staff to calibrate data from POCD devices and support lay users, even patients. Additionally, they have a team of IT professionals who can manage and maintain the technology infrastructure and ensure that the systems are secure and compliant with relevant regulations.

Organizations have access to a full range of digital technology for augmenting diagnostic tests and exams. Neural networks and machine learning models are deployed across all types of diagnostic tests and exams and data are integrated across functional areas to enable cross-disciplinary insights into multiple medical conditions (e.g., from pneumology to oncology and cardiology). POCD devices are deployed for remote diagnostic services across the ecosystem, even in patient homes. The technology infrastructure is scalable, reliable and secure and feeds into the rest of the processes of the healthcare delivery cycle. This can provide a structured and coordinated approach to diagnosis and can help ensure the best possible diagnostic outcomes.

3.2.3.3 *Preparing*

Organizations have a comprehensive and well-defined strategy in place for digitally preparing patients for different treatment options across their ecosystem. One of their key strategies is the use of electronic care planning and patient engagement tools. These tools allow healthcare providers to create individualized care plans for patients, and involve patients in the care planning process. For example, digital service providers can help healthcare providers integrate digital technologies into their preparation processes such as by providing expertise and support in the development of decision support systems and other tools that can help patients understand their treatment options and make informed decisions. Further, machine learning experts can provide AI chatbots for general queries before directing patients to specialized professionals. These ecosystem partnerships are defined with clear strategic goals and governance rules in place to achieve high value creation and capture in the preparing process. More importantly, by involving patients in the care planning process, they can better understand their needs and preferences, leading to more effective and efficient treatment. Patients can receive care planning and preparation without having to leave their homes, which can be particularly beneficial for patients with mobility issues or those who live in remote areas. Additionally, by using technology to facilitate collaboration and consultation among specialists, patients can receive a second opinion from a specialist without having to travel to a different location.

Organizations have staff members who are highly trained and skilled in the use of digital technology for preparing patients for different treatment options. There are psychologists and other specialized staff working closely with data scientists to collect and analyze data in real time, while providing targeted feedback to individual patients. There are dedicated leaders from clinical, data analytics and IT domains all of whom apply clear governance rules for handling sensitive patient queries, while ensuring that the systems are secure and compliant with relevant regulations.

Organizations have access to a full range of digital technology for preparing patients for different treatment options, including electronic care planning and patient engagement tools, EHRs, telemedicine and cloud-based systems. There are integrated services, including patient-facing platforms, virtual and augmented reality technologies, as well as AI-enabled chatbots. These services are integrated in a scalable, reliable and secure infrastructure. This can provide a consistent and structured approach to supporting and guiding patients and can help ensure the best possible health outcomes.

3.2.3.4   *Treating*

Organizations have a comprehensive and well-defined strategy in place for augmenting treatment options with digital technology across their ecosystem. One of the key strategies they use is the integration of robotic systems and minimally invasive surgical techniques. These technologies allow for more precise and accurate treatment, leading to improved patient outcomes and faster recovery times. Additionally, organizations with high digital maturity in treating use technology to facilitate collaboration and consultation among specialists. They use EHRs and telemedicine to share patient information and collaborate on treatment plans, regardless of their physical location. In addition, key strategic partners such as pharmaceutical and biotech companies can provide healthcare providers with access to the latest drugs and therapies that can support the treatment of patients. Finally, AI technology providers can provide AI systems to assist in treatment plans; this can be done by identifying the best treatment options for a patient's specific condition, and also by monitoring patients' progress and adjusting treatment plans if necessary. All of these strategic partnerships co-create value for patients by enabling more efficient and effective treatment, as well as improved continuity of care for patients.

Organizations have staff members who are highly trained and skilled in the use of digital technology for augmenting treatment options. They have a team of trained healthcare professionals who are able to use and interpret the data provided by the treatment technology. They also have a team of data analysts who can use data analytics to gain insights into population health, identify trends and patterns and improve the overall quality of care. Additionally, they have a team of IT professionals who can manage and maintain the technology infrastructure and ensure that the systems are secure and compliant with relevant regulations.

Organizations have access to a full range of digital technology for augmenting treatment options. Such technologies include robotic systems, minimally invasive surgical techniques, EHRs, telemedicine, cloud-based systems, AI systems developing personalized treatment plans, genomic systems and data analytics. These technologies allow organizations to perform more precise and accurate treatments, facilitate collaboration and consultation among specialists and improve the patient experience. The technology infrastructure is governed and architected for scale, reliability and security. This can provide a structured and coordinated approach to treatment and can help ensure the best possible treatment outcomes.

3.2.3.5   *Recovering*

Organizations have a comprehensive and well-defined strategy in place for providing rehabilitation and recovery for patients across their ecosystem. One of the key strategies is the use of augmented and virtual reality for rehabilitation. These technologies can improve the effectiveness and efficiency of physical therapy, making it more engaging for patients and easier for therapists to track progress. Key strategic partners such as medical device manufacturers can provide healthcare providers with advanced medical technologies such as rehabilitation robotics in combination with virtual reality systems to support the rehabilitation and recovery of patients. In addition, digital service providers can help healthcare providers integrate digital technologies in their recovering process.

Organizations have staff members who are highly trained and skilled in the use of digital technology for providing rehabilitation and recovery for patients. They have a team of trained healthcare professionals who are able to use and interpret the data provided by the recovery technology. They also have a team of data analysts who can use data analytics to gain insights into population health, identify trends and patterns and improve the overall quality of care. Additionally, they have a team of IT professionals who can manage and maintain the technology infrastructure and ensure that the systems are secure and compliant with relevant regulations.

Organizations have access to a full range of digital technology for providing rehabilitation and recovery for patients. telemedicine, remote monitoring, EHRs, augmented and virtual reality for rehabilitation and cloud-based systems. These technologies allow them to provide follow-up care and rehabilitation remotely, facilitate collaboration and consultation among specialists and improve the patient experience. They also have data analytics tools that can be used to gain insights into population health and improve the overall quality of care. Additionally, they have robust IT infrastructure that can manage and maintain these systems securely and compliant with relevant regulations. This can provide a structured and coordinated approach to supporting patients during this phase of their treatment and can help ensure the best possible recovery outcomes.

3.3   Becoming a Digital-First Organization

The discussion on digital maturity in the previous sections is meant to be used as an assessment blueprint. Healthcare organizations can use this assessment blueprint to identify where they stand on digital maturity across the five processes of the healthcare delivery cycle and the three dimensions of strategy, human and technology capabilities. By going through this exercise, incumbent organizations can begin to develop plans for transforming themselves into higher levels of digital maturity. New entrants can also use the assessment blueprint to craft comprehensive plans for becoming a digital-first organization.

A **digital-first organization** is not one that simply implements digital technologies to support non-digital processes. Rather, *a digital-first organization has a comprehensive digital strategy where people, processes, and structures are all digitally augmented, transforming the work environment.*[77]

A digital-first organization can compete with organizations with high digital maturity like the ones discussed above by continuously innovating new ways to use digital technology to improve patient outcomes, reduce costs and improve the overall quality of care. A digital-first organization invests in robust data management systems and continuously builds a team of data analysts to extract insights into health trends and patterns and improve the overall quality of healthcare services. Such organizations focus on providing personalized and patient-centric care by using smart sensors, wearable devices and such technology as remote monitoring and patient engagement tools while tapping on new advances in biotech and genomics research. Digital-first organizations foster collaboration and consultation among specialists, regardless of their physical location and have the ability to scale by leveraging digital platforms to accommodate more patients, more locations and more partners.

Examples of such digital-first organizations include Teladoc Health that provides remote, virtual medical consultations. It competes with traditional healthcare providers by offering more convenient and accessible healthcare services to patients and has been able to scale its services by partnering with national and private payers and employers. Teladoc Health has been able to outcompete incumbents by providing more convenient and accessible healthcare services to patients. It has experienced significant growth in its user base and revenue, with an expected 18.6 million visits and a total of 58 million US memberships in 2022, while its annual revenue is expected to hit $2,410 million.[78] Another example of a digital-first organization is Medopad[79] (recently acquired by Huma[80]), a UK-based startup, financed by the German pharmaceutical company Bayer, Hong Kong's NWS Holdings and Chicago's VC Healthbox, and working with Chinese firms Tencent and Ping An, among others. Modepad has grown its services to more than 27 million patients, across 3,000 hospitals and clinics.

Becoming a digital-first organization requires, first, understanding how value can be created across the five processes of the healthcare delivery cycle and developing a clear digital strategy that can improve patient outcomes, reduce costs and improve the overall quality of care. It also involves assessing the current state of technology across the healthcare sector and identifying the gaps that need to be filled in order to fully leverage technology to augment the key processes. Second, digital-first organizations need to build a team of digital experts, including healthcare professionals, IT professionals and data analysts, who can help to implement and manage the technology. They need to invest in training and development for all staff to ensure that they are able to fully leverage the technology across the five processes of the healthcare delivery cycle. Third, digital-first organizations need to look for partners and technology providers that can help to fill the gaps in the organization's technology stack. These partners should have experience working in healthcare and should have a proven track record of delivering results. Fourth, a competent team, in collaboration with teams from partner organizations, should take on the task of implementing and integrating the technology stack, making sure that it is secure and compliant with relevant regulations. Through the aforementioned steps, digital-first organizations need to continuously monitor and evaluate the success of the digital transformation by measuring the impact on patient outcomes, costs and overall quality of care. They need to use this data to make adjustments and continue to improve the technology stack.

New entrants and digital startups are not constrained by legacy systems and a workforce that lacks digital capabilities; thus, they have great opportunities to become digital-first organizations. However, they are constrained by means of financial resources and access to partners and customers that would allow them to speed up transformation. Incumbent organizations with strong user and partner bases can shift their services and transform their capabilities toward higher digital maturity. This constant race toward digital maturity, on the one hand, and the disruption that is brought by digital-first organizations, on the other, shape how ecosystems are formed and what role different organizations play in those. The next chapter examines in depth an ecosystem approach to digital transformation.

Notes

1 Poole, M.S. and Van de Ven, A.H., eds., 2004. *Handbook of Organizational Change and Innovation.* Oxford University Press, Oxford, UK; Burke, W.W., 2017. *Organization Change: Theory and Practice.* Sage Publications, London UK.; Peters, T.J. and Waterman, R.H., 1982. *In Search of Excellence: Lessons from America's Best-Run Companies.* Harper Business, New York, USA; Collins, J.C. and Porras, J., 1994. *Built to last: Successful Habits of Visionary Companies.* Random House, New York, USA; Welch, J. and Byrne, J.A., 2003. *Jack: Straight from the Gut.* Business Plus, New York, USA.

2 Foster, R. and Kaplan, S., 2001. *Creative Destruction: Why Companies That Are Built to Last Underperform the Market – And How to Successfully Transform Them.* Currency, New York, USA.

3 Ibid.

4 Ibid. p. 16.

5 Pascale, R., Milleman, M. and Gioja, L., 2001. *Surfing the Edge of Chaos: The Laws of Nature and the New Laws of Business.* Texere, New York, USA.

6 Burke, W.W., 2017. *Organization Change: Theory and Practice.* Sage Publications, London UK.

7 Porter, M. 1998. *On Competition.* Harvard Business Review Press, Boston USA.

8 Porter, M.E. and Teisberg, E.O., 2006. *Redefining health care: creating value-based competition on results.* Harvard Business Review Press, Boston USA.

9 Topol, E., 2015. *The patient will see you now: the future of medicine is in your hands.* Basic Books, New York, USA.

10 Hou, Y.C.C., Yu, H.C., Martin, R., Schenker-Ahmed, N.M., Hicks, M., Cirulli, E.T., Cohen, I.V., Jonsson, T.J., Heister, R., Napier, L. and Swisher, C.L., 2018. Precision medicine advancements using whole genome sequencing, noninvasive whole body imaging, and functional diagnostics. *bioRxiv*, p. 497560; also see https://humanlongevity.com/ (previously called HealthNucleus). https://www.biorxiv.org/content/10.1101/497560v1

11 See Sian Jones, Head of Service Improvement at Bristol Clinical Commissioning Group explain this monitoring service here https://www.kingsfund.org.uk/audio-video/sian-jones-exploration-large-scale-implementation-telehealth-monitoring-bristol

12 Y Yang, Z., Huang, Y., Jiang, Y., Sun, Y., Zhang, Y.J. and Luo, P., 2018. Clinical assistant diagnosis for electronic medical record based on convolutional neural network. *Scientific Reports*, 8(1), p. 6329; Razavian, N., Marcus, J., and Sontag, D., 2016. Multi-task prediction of disease onsets from longitudinal lab tests. *PMLR*, 56, pp. 73–100.

13 Plevniak, K., Campbell, M., Myers, T., Hodges, A. and He, M., 2016. 3D printed auto-mixing chip enables rapid smartphone diagnosis of anemia. *Biomicrofluidics*, 10(5), p. 054113; Barbosa, A.I., Gehlot, P., Sidapra, K., Edwards, A.D. and Reis, N.M., 2015. Portable smartphone quantitation of prostate specific antigen (PSA) in a fluoropolymer microfluidic device. *Biosensors and Bioelectronics*, 70, pp. 5–14; Laksanasopin, T., Guo, T.W., Nayak, S., Sridhara, A.A., Xie, S., Olowookere, O.O., Cadinu, P., Meng, F., Chee, N.H., Kim, J. and Chin, C.D., 2015. A smartphone dongle for diagnosis of infectious diseases at the point of care. *Science Translational Medicine*, 7(273), pp. 273re1–273re1.

14 Sarioglu, A.F., Aceto, N., Kojic, N., Donaldson, M.C., Zeinali, M., Hamza, B., Engstrom, A., Zhu, H., Sundaresan, T.K., Miyamoto, D.T. and Luo, X., 2015. A microfluidic device for label-free, physical capture of circulating tumor cell clusters. *Nature Methods*, 12(7), pp. 685–691.

15 See https://www.moorfields.nhs.uk/content/latest-updates-deepmind-health

16 Howard-Anderson, J., Ganz, P.A., Bower, J.E. and Stanton, A.L., 2012. Quality of life, fertility concerns, and behavioral health outcomes in younger breast cancer survivors: a systematic review. *Journal of the National Cancer Institute*, 104(5), pp. 386–405.

17 Koç, Z., Kaplan, E. and Tanrıverdi, D., 2022. The effectiveness of telehealth programs on the mental health of women with breast cancer: a systematic review. *Journal of Telemedicine and Telecare*, 0(0)p. 1357633×X211069663. https://journals.sagepub.com/doi/abs/10.1177/1357633X211069663

18 See https://insilico.com/platform and https://www.benevolent.com/what-we-do

19 Topol, E. 2019. *Deep Medicine: How Artificial Intelligence Can Make Healthcare Human Again.* Basic Books. New York, USA.

20 Constantinides, P. and Fitzmaurice, D.A., 2018. Artificial intelligence in cardiology: applications, benefits and challenges. *The British Journal of Cardiology, 25*, pp. 1–3.

21 Vávra, P., Roman, J., Zonča, P., Ihnát, P., Němec, M., Kumar, J., Habib, N. and El-Gendi, A., 2017. Recent development of augmented reality in surgery: a review. *Journal of Healthcare Engineering, 2017*; Pulijala, Y., Ma, M., Pears, M., Peebles, D. and Ayoub, A., 2018. Effectiveness of immersive virtual reality in surgical training—a randomized control trial. *Journal of Oral and Maxillofacial Surgery, 76*(5), pp. 1065–1072.

22 Uppot, R.N., Laguna, B., McCarthy, C.J., De Novi, G., Phelps, A., Siegel, E. and Courtier, J., 2019. Implementing virtual and augmented reality tools for radiology education and training, communication, and clinical care. *Radiology, 291*(3), pp. 570–580; Gibby, J.T., Swenson, S.A., Cvetko, S., Rao, R. and Javan, R., 2019. Head-mounted display augmented reality to guide pedicle screw placement utilizing computed tomography. *International Journal of Computer Assisted Radiology and Surgery, 14*(3), pp. 525–535.

23 Burke, J.W., McNeill, M.D.J., Charles, D.K., Morrow, P.J., Crosbie, J.H. and McDonough, S.M., 2010 . Augmented reality games for upper-limb stroke rehabilitation. In *2010 Second International Conference on Games and Virtual Worlds for Serious Applications* (pp. 75–78). IEEE, Braga, Portugal.

24 Mousavi Hondori, H. and Khademi, M., 2014. A review on technical and clinical impact of microsoft kinect on physical therapy and rehabilitation. *Journal of Medical Engineering, pp.* 1–6; Garcia-Agundez, A., Folkerts, A.K., Konrad, R., Caserman, P., Tregel, T., Goosses, M., Göbel, S. and Kalbe, E., 2019. Recent advances in rehabilitation for Parkinson's disease with exergames: a systematic review. *Journal of Neuroengineering and Rehabilitation, 16*(1), pp. 1–17.

25 Gardner, H.E., 1995. *Leading Minds: An Anatomy of Leadership.* Basic Books, New York, USA.

26 Whetten, D.A., 2006. Albert and Whetten revisited: Strengthening the concept of organizational identity. *Journal of Management Inquiry, 15*(3), pp. 219–234; Gioia, D.A., Schultz, M. and Corley, K.G., 2000. Organizational identity, image, and adaptive instability. *Academy of Management Review, 25*(1), pp. 63–81; Livengood, R.S., and Reger, R.K. 2010. That's our turf! Identity domains and competitive dynamics. *Academy of Management Review, 35*, pp. 48–66.

27 Yoffie, D.B. and Cusumano, M.A., 2015. *Strategy Rules: Five Timeless Lessons from Bill Gates, Andy Grove, and Steve Jobs.* Harper Collins, New York USA.

28 Ibid.

29 Berry, L.L. and Seltman, K.D., 2008. *Management Lessons from Mayo Clinic.* McGraw-Hill Professional Publishing, New York, USA.

30 Ibid. p. 20.

31 Roberts, B.W., Walton, K.E. and Viechtbauer, W., 2006. Patterns of mean-level change in personality traits across the life course: a meta-analysis of longitudinal studies. *Psychological Bulletin, 132*(1), p. 1; Choi, M., 2011. Employees' attitudes toward organizational change: a literature review. *Human Resource Management, 50*(4), pp. 479–500.; Weick, K.E. and Quinn, R.E., 1999. Organizational change and development. *Annual Review of Psychology, 50*(1), pp. 361–386.

32 Ashforth, B.K. and Saks, A.M., 1996. Socialization tactics: Longitudinal effects on newcomer adjustment. *Academy of Management Journal, 39*(1), pp. 149–178.; Pratt, M.G., Rockmann, K.W. and Kaufmann, J.B., 2006. Constructing professional identity: the role of work and identity learning cycles in the customization of identity among medical residents. *Academy of Management Journal, 49*(2), pp. 235–262; Kristof-Brown, A.L., Zimmerman, R.D. and Johnson, E.C., 2005. Consequences of individuals' fit at work: a meta-analysis of person–job, person–organization, person–group, and person–supervisor fit. *Personnel Psychology, 58*(2), pp. 281–342.

33 John, O.P., Robins, R.W. and Pervin, L.A. eds., 2010. *Handbook of Personality: Theory and Research.* Guilford Press, New York, USA.

34 Lubinski, D., 2000. Scientific and social significance of assessing individual differences: sinking shafts at a few critical points. *Annual Review of Psychology, 51*(1), pp. 405–444.

35 Tripsas, M., 2009. Technology, identity, and inertia through the lens of "The Digital Photography Company". *Organization Science, 20*(2), pp. 441–460; Mishra, A.N., Anderson, C., Angst, C.M. and Agarwal, R., 2012. Electronic health records assimilation and physician identity evolution: an identity theory perspective. *Information Systems Research, 23*(3-part-1), pp. 738–760; Carter, M., Petter, S., Grover, V. and Thatcher, J.B., 2020.

Information technology identity: a key determinant of IT feature and exploratory usage. *MIS Quarterly*, 44(3), pp. 983–1021.

36 Mishra, A.N., Anderson, C., Angst, C.M. and Agarwal, R., 2012. Electronic health records assimilation and physician identity evolution: an identity theory perspective. *Information Systems Research*, 23(3-part-1), pp.738–760.

37 See recent report by the Boston Consulting Group on the digital maturity of different organizations by industry. https://www.bcg.com/publications/2022/digital-transformation-efforts-report

38 See for example the Global Health Observatory by the World Health Organization https://www.who.int/data/gho/data/themes/topics/topic-details/GHO/world-health-statistics

39 Consultancy firms like PwC produce reports on such global issues as social determinants of health that are meant to offer broad guidance to healthcare providers and national payers. See https://www.pwc.com/gx/en/industries/healthcare/publications/social-determinants-of-health.html

40 See recent report by van der Kleij, R.M., Kasteleyn, M.J., Meijer, E., Bonten, T.N., Houwink, E.J., Teichert, M., van Luenen, S., Vedanthan, R., Evers, A., Car, J. and Pinnock, H., 2019. SERIES: eHealth in primary care. Part 1: concepts, conditions and challenges. *European Journal of General Practice*, 25(4), pp. 179–189.

41 Kleinberger, T., Becker, M., Ras, E., Holzinger, A. and Müller, P., 2007, July. Ambient intelligence in assisted living: enable elderly people to handle future interfaces. In *International Conference on Universal Access in Human-Computer Interaction* (pp. 103–112). Springer, Berlin, Heidelberg.

42 Sapci, A.H. and Sapci, H.A., 2019. Innovative assisted living tools, remote monitoring technologies, artificial intelligence-driven solutions, and robotic systems for aging societies: systematic review. *JMIR Aging*, 2(2), p. e15429.

43 KPMG, "The Healthcare Diagnostics Value Game" https://assets.kpmg/content/dam/kpmg/xx/pdf/2018/07/the-healthcare-diagnostics-value-game.pdf

44 See https://americanhealthimaging.com/blog/why-mri-cost-much-hospital/ and https://heartlandimagingcenters.com/2021/03/19/why-are-mris-so-expensive-at-hospitals/

45 Quinn, M., Forman, J., Harrod, M., Winter, S., Fowler, K.E., Krein, S.L., Gupta, A., Saint, S., Singh, H. and Chopra, V., 2019. Electronic health records, communication, and data sharing: challenges and opportunities for improving the diagnostic process. *Diagnosis*, 6(3), pp. 241–248.

46 Silver, J.K. and Baima, J., 2013. Cancer prehabilitation: an opportunity to decrease treatment-related morbidity, increase cancer treatment options, and improve physical and psychological health outcomes. *American Journal of Physical Medicine & Rehabilitation*, 92(8), pp. 715–727.

47 Aziz, K.T., Nayar, S.K., LaPorte, D.M., Ingari, J.V. and Giladi, A.M., 2022. Impact of missing data on identifying risk factors for postoperative complications in hand surgery. *Hand*, 17(6), pp. 1257–1263.

48 de Melo Santos, T.T., dos Santos Andrade, L.S., de Oliveira, M.E.C., Gomes, K.A.L., de Oliveira, T.A. and Weller, M., 2020. Availability of diagnostic services and their impact on patient flow in two Brazilian referral centres of breast cancer treatment. *Asian Pacific Journal of Cancer Prevention: APJCP*, 21(2), p. 317.

49 Ibid.

50 McGrath, S.P., McGovern, K.M., Perreard, I.M., Huang, V., Moss, L.B. and Blike, G.T., 2021. Inpatient respiratory arrest associated with sedative and analgesic medications: impact of continuous monitoring on patient mortality and severe morbidity. *Journal of Patient Safety*, 17(8), p. 557.

51 Lowres, N., Mulcahy, G., Jin, K., Gallagher, R., Neubeck, L. and Freedman, B., 2018. Incidence of postoperative atrial fibrillation recurrence in patients discharged in sinus rhythm after cardiac surgery: a systematic review and meta-analysis. *Interactive Cardiovascular and Thoracic Surgery*, 26(3), pp. 504–511.

52 See listing on the GOV.UK website https://find-and-update.company-information.service.gov.uk/company/03891401

53 See a review of such IoT systems in Hassanalieragh, M., Page, A., Soyata, T., Sharma, G., Aktas, M., Mateos, G., and Andreescu, S., 2015. Health monitoring and management using Internet-of-Things (IoT) sensing with cloud-based processing: Opportunities and challenges. In *2015 IEEE International Conference on Services Computing* (pp. 285–292). IEEE, New York, USA.

54 KPMG, "The Healthcare Diagnostics Value Game" https://assets.kpmg/content/dam/kpmg/xx/pdf/2018/07/the-healthcare-diagnostics-value-game.pdf
55 Ibid.
56 https://www.rcr.ac.uk/posts/new-rcr-census-shows-nhs-needs-nearly-2000-more-radiologists
57 Ibid.
58 https://www.rsna.org/news/2022/may/Global-Radiologist-Shortage
59 https://www.diagnosticimaging.com/view/to-remain-a-technology-leader-radiology-must-train-residents-in-machine-learning
60 See https://www.patientslikeme.com/about/partners
61 PatientsLikeMe was acquired by UnitedHealth Group in 2019 https://www.mobihealthnews.com/content/unitedhealth-group-acquires-patientslikeme
62 Eccleston, C., Fisher, E., Liikkanen, S., Sarapohja, T., Stenfors, C., Jääskeläinen, S.K., Rice, A.S., Mattila, L., Blom, T. and Bratty, J.R., 2022. A prospective, double-blind, pilot, randomized, controlled trial of an "embodied" virtual reality intervention for adults with low back pain. *Pain*, 163(9), pp. 1700–1715.
63 https://www.xr.health/product-new/
64 Ibid.
65 https://fundamentalsurgery.com/platform/
66 Bjarnason-Wehrens, B., McGee, H., Zwisler, A.D., Piepoli, M.F., Benzer, W., Schmid, J.P., Dendale, P., Pogosova, N.G.V., Zdrenghea, D., Niebauer, J. and Mendes, M., 2010. Cardiac rehabilitation in Europe: results from the European cardiac rehabilitation inventory survey. *European Journal of Preventive Cardiology*, 17(4), pp. 410–418; Beatty, A.L., Truong, M., Schopfer, D.W., Shen, H., Bachmann, J.M. and Whooley, M.A., 2018. Geographic variation in cardiac rehabilitation participation in Medicare and Veterans Affairs populations: opportunity for improvement. *Circulation*, 137(18), pp. 1899–1908.
67 Thomas, R.J., Beatty, A.L., Beckie, T.M., Brewer, L.C., Brown, T.M., Forman, D.E., Franklin, B.A., Keteyian, S.J., Kitzman, D.W., Regensteiner, J.G. and Sanderson, B.K., 2019. Home-based cardiac rehabilitation: a scientific statement from the American Association of Cardiovascular and Pulmonary Rehabilitation, the American Heart Association, and the American College of Cardiology. *Circulation*, 140(1), pp. e69-e89; National Institute for Health and Care Excellence. Chronic heart failure in adults: diagnosis and management. NICE Guideline NG106. London: NICE, 2018. https://www.nice.org.uk/guidance/ng106
68 https://inmotionvr.com/
69 https://mindmaze.com/about/
70 https://www.healthcareitnews.com/vmware/cleveland-clinic-leveraging-technology-transform-patient-and-clinician-experience
71 https://newsnetwork.mayoclinic.org/discussion/entering-the-digital-front-door-to-a-better-health-care-experience/
72 https://www.royalmarsden.nhs.uk/green-plan-digital-transformation
73 See report on China's "Internet Hospitals" by Deloitte https://www2.deloitte.com/content/dam/Deloitte/cn/Documents/life-sciences-health-care/deloitte-cn-lshc-internet-hospitals-in-china-the-new-step-into-digital-healthcare-en-210315.pdf
74 https://opengovasia.com/journey-towards-revolutionising-healthcare-at-seoul-national-university-bundang-hospital/
75 https://www.karolinska.se/en/karolinska-university-hospital/Innovation/innovation-partnership/hpe/
76 https://www.mobihealthnews.com/news/emea/uae-s-mulk-healthcare-launches-global-e-hospital
77 Baskerville, R., Myers, M.D. and Yoo, Y., 2020. Digital first: the ontological reversal and new challenges for IS research. *MIS Quarterly*, 44(2), pp. 509–523.
78 99https://ir.teladochealth.com/news-and-events/investor-news/press-release-details/2022/Teladoc-Health-Reports-Third-Quarter-2022-Results/default.aspx
79 https://medopad.com/
80 https://huma.com/

Part 2

Digital Transformation across Healthcare Ecosystems

Part 2 is the core of the book providing a detailed discussion of the ecosystem approach to digital transformation. It discusses how organizations can develop their own ecosystem or become a partner in other ecosystems. This approach is not simply about technology. It is about collaborating on complex problems and finding innovative solutions, establishing governance mechanisms for managing risks and resolving collective action problems, and building joint value propositions that generate virtuous value creation opportunities for all ecosystem actors.

First, Chapter 4 lays out a framework of how organizations can digitally transform their services across an ecosystem, including how to define their digital transformation problem, clarify their incentives and activities, but also how to develop an innovation and adoption plan in collaboration with their partners, while governing associated risks. The chapter draws heavily on the example of the Siemens Healthineers' "teamplay digital health platform", which enables diverse organizations, from hospitals to diagnostic centers, to benefit from a vendor-agnostic, modular infrastructure and digital applications provided by third-party complementors on demand. The chapter discusses both the opportunities and collective action problems that may emerge in such ecosystems and also provides ways of effectively managing those while ensuring the sustainability and growth of the ecosystem.

Chapter 5 discusses how healthcare organizations can form ecosystems on blockchain infrastructures. This chapter describes how blockchain infrastructures work, how transactions take place and how they enable distributed data governance. It then provides a discussion of use cases of blockchain infrastructures in healthcare provided by PharmaLedger, focusing on recruiting patients and achieving informed consent in clinical trials, and achieving trusted transactions through electronic product information in pharmaceutical supply chains. The chapter concludes by discussing the co-innovation and co-adoption challenges of the use of blockchain infrastructures in healthcare.

Chapter 6 discusses ways by which healthcare organizations can form ecosystems on federated learning infrastructures. The chapter describes how cloud computing works, before exploring data virtualization and federated learning infrastructures. It then discusses two use cases of federated learning in healthcare ecosystems, one in medical imaging used during the COVID-19 pandemic and one in genomics research hosted on the Lifebit platform. The chapter concludes by discussing the co-innovation and co-adoption challenges of the use of data virtualization in healthcare.

DOI: 10.4324/9781032619569-5

4   An Ecosystem Approach to Digital Transformation

Chapter 1 has already discussed how on-demand, digital platforms such as Doximity, Doctor Care Anywhere and Ping An Good Doctor but also home care platforms such as Doccla[1] have disrupted healthcare services. Healthcare service providers dependent on geographical boundaries are at risk of being left out without any patients to cater to. Similarly, new startups developing embodied, wearable and mobile devices are disrupting traditional relationships between patients, service providers and other ecosystem actors. The advent of genomic technologies such as next-generation whole genome sequencing and nanotechnologies, combined with an increased interest in precision medicine, has pushed for the development of such devices beyond traditional modalities of care.[2] Such digital and biotechnology innovations are capitalizing on the rising costs of more traditional modalities of care, high waiting times and the burnout of healthcare professionals, as discussed in Chapter 2. Most importantly, such innovations are disrupting existing value propositions by incumbents, by breaking established organizational boundaries. Similarly, health insurers are the most disrupted given that their products are directly associated with cost scale economies. Any big actor with the ability to support such cost scale economies can disrupt incumbent health insurers' position. For example, Ping An Insurance, China's largest insurer by market value, has, since COVID-19 struck, made significant investments in healthcare technology that aim to fill resource gaps in China's national health system, while disrupting incumbents in digital health.[3] In the USA, Amazon has entered the pharmaceutical supply sector after acquiring PillPack, allowing Amazon Prime members to access free two-day delivery of orders with savings of up to 80 percent off generic and 40 percent off branded medications when not paying using insurance.[4] These examples show the disruption risk that incumbents could be facing if they only look inwards for their digital transformation.

Healthcare organizations are faced with complex problems that will often necessitate coordinating multiple actors and their unique resources and capabilities to develop more cost-effective, safe and innovative solutions. The complexity of healthcare service provision requires healthcare organizations to start exploring new value propositions with other ecosystem actors in order to synergistically combine resources and capabilities that can scale, that can have a wider scope than if staying within organizational boundaries and that can exert higher levels of influence on other ecosystem actors to shape digital transformation with long-term impact. These are key conditions for adopting an ecosystem approach to digital transformation. Certainly, the digital maturity of each organization will define its role in the ecosystem. Organizations with high digital maturity are in a better position to orchestrate ecosystems, whereas organizations with low and medium digital maturity can become partners, some with a more strategic role than others.

DOI: 10.4324/9781032619569-6

This chapter provides an ecosystem approach to digital transformation. It elaborates on how organizations can build their own ecosystem and orchestrate the activities of others, but also how they can participate in other ecosystems. The chapter provides a detailed framework of how organizations can digitally transform their services across an ecosystem, including how to define their digital transformation problem, clarify their incentives and activities, but also how to develop an innovation and adoption plan in collaboration with their partners, while governing associated risks.

4.1 Mapping the Ecosystem

First, organizations need to identify which ecosystem to participate in and what are the co-dependencies with other ecosystem actors. Along the lines of what was observed with manufacturing supply chains during COVID-19, such mapping includes negotiating greater visibility into the current state and future plans of other actors' activities.[5] This involves understanding what each actor brings to the ecosystem, whether that includes resources to realize a strategy or human or technological capabilities, but also what each actor gains from the ecosystem. These co-dependencies help define the necessary incentives for synergistic combinations to emerge in relation to the costs to be incurred and benefits to be captured by each actor. The benefits include the production and consumption of services, access to new markets through affiliated partners, access to data and many more. For example, digital platforms such as Doctor Care Anywhere and Doccla can partner with primary care doctors who can provide services to patients on demand, minimizing patient waiting times, as well as travel costs, and maximizing convenience, while at the same time, potentially also impacting quality through peer recommendations. Thus, ecosystem actors, rather than being stuck in individual sets of relationships, each fraught with their own risks, can benefit from a greater set of options. The benefit is amplified when the value for individual actors spills over other actors – more patients attract more primary care doctors, in turn attracting even additional services such as specialized care for chronic disease patients.

In exchange, however, actors need to let go of some control over previously hierarchically managed resources and capabilities because this would immediately kill incentives for collaboration with other ecosystem actors. In an ecosystem, different actors multilaterally coordinate their efforts to synergistically combine resources and capabilities. Unlike more supply-driven forms of organizing innovation, in ecosystems, the type and quality of services, as well as the prices are left to vary, and to be designed as a function of the capabilities of different ecosystem actors.[6] This is the fundamental structural feature that makes ecosystem interactions strategically distinct. Ecosystem actors are bound together through common standards, rules and interfaces that are often set by a focal organization. However, ecosystem actors retain some control and claims over their resources and capabilities. In this way, the ecosystem can constantly grow, allowing more actors to join, while bringing in new services that can help attract yet new customers.

One successful example of how an organization can benefit from an ecosystem approach to digital transformation is Zwanger-Pesiri Radiology, an outpatient radiology practice based in the metropolitan New York area on Long Island. Zwanger-Pesiri Radiology operates across 33 locations with 70+ radiologists and 1,300 employees. They do approximately 4,300 exams a day, 800 of which are MRI scans, 1,000 are ultrasound scans and another 1,000 are X-ray scans. Additional exams include CT scans, mammographies, dexa and other procedures. Zwanger-Pesiri Radiology faced a number of challenges to try and grow the practice. First, they faced the challenge of exchanging data between locations and domain experts that was not streamlined, dependable and robust to allow information officers to monitor levels of service. Second, they were faced with non-interoperability between some of their varied data sources, which again inhibited an understanding of the level and quality of services being offered to patients and institutional customers. Finally, they used different technology solutions provided by different vendors that did not integrate very well with their core systems.

To address these challenges and digitally transform their practice, Zwanger-Pesiri Radiology partnered with Siemens Healthineers taking advantage of their "teamplay digital health platform", which enables diverse organizations to benefit from cloud computing services and digital applications on demand.[7] By moving their digital infrastructure on the cloud, Zwanger-Pesiri Radiology achieved interoperability between varied data sources and technology solutions through the API provided by Siemens Healthineers. More importantly, the digital services offered on the teamplay platform are compliant with regulations such as GDPR and HIPAA and security protocols managed through Microsoft Azure data centers. Zwanger-Pesiri Radiology now enjoys cloud-orchestrated updates for digital applications running on Siemens medical devices. This accelerates opportunities for demand economies of scale and scope. In addition, Zwanger-Pesiri Radiology now has access to AI-powered analytics through the teamplay platform that allows the practice to optimize operations.

Specifically, the team at Zwanger-Pesiri Radiology have been working closely with the team from Siemens Healthineers to adapt the AI-Rad Companion. This is an AI-powered, augmented workflow solution that allows Zwanger-Pesiri Radiology to reduce the burden of work for their radiologists, while also increasing their diagnostic precision when interpreting medical images. For example, the AI-Rad Companion Chest CT can detect and highlight lung nodules, segment them, define the volume, and calculate the maximum 2D and 3D diameters and tumor burden.[8] Cinematic and other types of rendering can add clarity to the location of a detected lung nodule, making it easier for the referring physician to get a clear picture of the nodule location within the lung. These and other features such as recognizing coronary calcium and measuring the aorta and vertebrae bodies are all delivered on demand via the cloud. More importantly, the algorithms and the machine learning models powering the AI-Rad Companion workflow solutions are constantly being updated and improved based on images and diagnostic decisions taken not just at Zwanger-Pesiri Radiology, but across 6,500 connected ecosystem actors, 32,000 connected systems in more than 60 countries with more than 10 million patient records.[9]

Zwanger-Pesiri Radiology is now part of the Siemens Healthineers' ecosystem orchestrated by Siemens through the teamplay digital health platform. This ecosystem provides a wide set of value propositions for the different ecosystem actors, including the healthcare service providers, and a growing base of complementors and patients. Table 4.1 summarizes these value propositions, which are discussed below in more detail.

The primary value proposition for ecosystem orchestrators like Siemens Healthineers is the potential to innovate on a scale and scope that is inconceivable if pursued independently by a single organization. Instead of itself attempting to innovate new digital health services in diverse domains, the ecosystem orchestrator can develop a digital platform and distribute innovation to large numbers of complementors. This allows the ecosystem orchestrator to organize an application marketplace based on standard interfaces such as API. Siemens Healthineers currently offers such a marketplace with more

Table 4.1 Value Propositions for Ecosystem Actors

Ecosystem Actors	Value Propositions: What Each Actor Gains from the Ecosystem
Ecosystem Orchestrator (e.g., Siemens Healthineers)	• Achieve distributed innovation across ecosystem actors • Share risk of digital innovation with ecosystem complementors • Share modular and scalable infrastructure resources • Maximize utilization of medical devices • Generate new digital services as add-ons to medical devices from data-driven insights gained from ecosystem partners and complementors • Capture long-tail markets across digital health service modalities • Gain larger market share and achieve competitive sustainability
Ecosystem Actors (professional users) (e.g., healthcare service providers such as hospitals and diagnostic centers)	• Avoid capital investments and gain access to a modular and scalable infrastructure and software deployment • Establish technological interoperability using a vendor-agnostic platform • Achieve data service compliance with established interoperability, privacy and security standards • Gain access to digital health solutions that are data-driven and AI-enabled from a curated marketplace • Benefit from data-driven insights from other ecosystem actors • Improve operational and diagnostic efficiencies • Benefit from spillover innovation from complementors • Benefit from lower search and transaction costs
Ecosystem Actors (complementors) (e.g., app developers, data aggregators, biobanks)	• Avoid capital investments and gain access to a standardized infrastructure through a set of API, while sharpening core competencies and internal research and development • Benefit from faster and wider market access • Benefit from lower search, transaction and delivery costs
Ecosystem Actors (users) Patients	• Gain wider and more convenient access to high-quality digital health services at relatively lower costs • Benefit from precision medicine

than 50 applications from selected developers.[10] Just like other application marketplaces such as the Apple App Store and the Google Play Store, the Siemens Healthineers' marketplace enables third-party complementors to innovate new applications that can be marketed on the teamplay platform for other ecosystem actors such as hospitals and diagnostic centers. The app marketplace can, thus, generate value creating interactions between complementors and healthcare service providers kickstarting network effects between the two sides.[11] Positive network effects can generate economies of scale and scope for the digital platform ecosystem such as building a larger user base of healthcare service providers adopting applications from complementors, as well as more domain-specific applications being developed to accommodate diverse needs. The more the network of users and complementors grows, the more valuable the ecosystem becomes for all involved. In this effort, the ecosystem orchestrator shares the financial and technical risk of innovation with the complementors. Therefore, unlike traditional product development, the costs and risks of developing new applications are distributed between the ecosystem orchestrator and the complementors. These complementors are driven by the hunger to succeed, with the prospects of large payoffs if they do. Complementors can therefore bolster the ecosystem's marketplace's competitive advantage purely by pursuing their self-interest (but only if governance is done right, as discussed later in the chapter).

In addition to this, Siemens Healthineers has an opportunity to maximize the utilization of their physical assets, their medical devices, that are already being used by their customers. Siemens Healthineers like other medical device manufacturers such as Philips, GE Healthcare and Samsung Medison are asset-heavy companies that have traditionally relied on the sales of their assets to healthcare service providers, while adding service costs for maintenance and support. Through an ecosystem approach, these medical device manufacturers can now use their medical assets as data-oriented digital platforms. As discussed above, Siemens Healthineers offers data-driven, AI-enabled workflow systems delivered through their teamplay platform. These workflow systems integrate with the medical devices that are physically located in different healthcare service providers' premises. They can, thus, maximize the utilization of their physical assets with value-added digital services developed by Siemens Healthineers in-house or by third-party complementors.

These value-added digital services enable the ecosystem orchestrator to capture long-tail markets – i.e., markets that are so different from their typical customer that relatively small incremental quantities of a product or service can be sold if the ecosystem orchestrator catered to that market on its own.[12] Usually, single organizations can only focus on the needs of their mass market in conceiving new products and services, because it is unviable for them to develop resources and capabilities to serve multiple other markets. However, long-tail markets with highly specialized and uncommon needs (relative to the mass market) can collectively add up to a substantial lost opportunity, often exceeding that of the mass market. For example, one of the third-party complementors on the teamplay platform is AMRA, whose cloud-based analysis service, AMRA Researcher "transforms images from a rapid whole body MRI scan into precise, 3D-volumetric fat and muscle measurements".[13] This application has already been adopted by healthcare service providers such as Human Longevity – discussed in Chapter 1 – that are focused on precision medicine services to patients. By developing a digital platform with a marketplace, Siemens Healthineers is in a position to capture such long-tail markets without having to attempt to create products and services for them. Instead, third-party app developers are more likely to find these long-tail markets lucrative enough to pursue using Siemens Healthineers' teamplay platform. The ecosystem orchestrator can therefore penetrate many long-tail markets through a digital platform, without bearing the direct costs or risks of doing so.

A final value proposition for ecosystem orchestrators is to increase their competitive sustainability. By offering value-added digital services on top of their successful physical assets, Siemens Healthineers increases the value of their ecosystem to both healthcare service providers and third-party app developers. Once a virtuous cycle of value co-creation begins, ecosystems can be difficult to overpower because a competitor would not only have to deliver a better price-to-performance ratio but would also have to build a user base, while at the same time incentivizing complementors to join. Organizations such as Siemens Healthineers that already offer compelling physical products such as their MRI and CT scanners are in a perfect position to become ecosystem orchestrators and overcome the chicken-and-egg dilemma of building the two sides in a digital platform.[14] They already have one side on board, the healthcare service providers, so they can easily attract the other side, the complementors. Once, at least two sides join, a digital platform can expand to multiple sides such as data biobanks, researchers and payers, thus expanding the value propositions offered by the ecosystem.

For healthcare service providers a core value proposition offered by the Siemens Healthineers teamplay platform is gaining access to a scalable and flexible infrastructure and software deployment. In conventional digital transformation projects, healthcare service providers would usually have to incur high capital investment costs to build or outsource the development and maintenance of a physical infrastructure and software applications. By opting for a cloud computing service solution, healthcare service providers reduce the time, effort and resources needed to drive digital transformation. By not building the infrastructure themselves or through technology vendors offering standalone, proprietary solutions, healthcare service providers can avoid falling victims of opportunistic behavior by vendors, lock-in and high switching costs. They can also make an effort to constantly stay relevant in the market by searching for the latest digital solutions. Instead, by opting for an ecosystem approach through a digital platform, healthcare service providers can quickly establish technological interoperability between the systems required for their different service modalities while using a vendor-agnostic platform, as in the case of Zwanger-Pesiri Radiology. They can also achieve data service compliance with established interoperability standards such as DICOM, Hl7 and FHIR, while at the same time meeting privacy and security regulations like GDPR and HIPAA. As discussed in Chapter 2, many healthcare service providers struggle to keep up to pace with new regulations and technical standards, when they should be focusing primarily on their service outcomes. By opting for a vendor-agnostic platform and letting the ecosystem orchestrator and its technology partners worry about all that complexity, healthcare service providers can focus on their core competencies.

In addition, healthcare service providers can gain access to digital health solutions that are data-driven and AI-enabled from a curated marketplace and, thus, benefit from data-driven insights from other ecosystem actors.[15] This is where the power of the ecosystem approach to digital transformation lies: the ability to co-create value in co-opetition[16] with other ecosystem actors. By joining the Siemens Healthineers' teamplay platform, healthcare service providers not only benefit from horizontal digital capabilities that other technology vendors offer but also benefit from vertical capabilities in domain expertise from value-added applications provided by complementors. They also learn from data-driven insights generated in other, potentially competing healthcare service providers, as those are integrated in updated versions of the AI-enabled workflow solutions. These additional capabilities enable healthcare service providers to improve operational and diagnostic efficiencies in multiple modalities from interventional angiography to computed tomography and molecular imaging.

Intra-platform competition among complements and inter-platform competition among competing digital platform ecosystems deliver a faster rate of innovation that is likely to benefit ecosystem actors such as healthcare service providers the most. Rival complements compete for these providers' attention. Similarly, rival digital platform ecosystems compete with each other to attract more healthcare service providers. This competition generates innovation spillovers while increasing quality for the providers. Finally, digital platform ecosystems can potentially reduce these providers' search costs, by curating competing complements such as screening and certifying them before they appear on the marketplace, like Siemens Healthineers does for its third-party app developers. Digital platform ecosystems can also reduce the costs incurred by the providers during their transactions with complementors through transaction and exchange mechanisms. Siemens Healthineers' teamplay platform, for example, offers different pricing models from one-time payments, pay-per-use or subscription models based on capital or operational expenditures.

For ecosystem complementors, a digital platform ecosystem provides a standardized infrastructure and resources such as software development kits (SDK) and API, as well as development environments upon which they can build their work. For example, Siemens Healthineers offers complementors their syngo.via OpenApps environment to develop and test their applications before these become integrated on the teamplay platform. This allows thousands of complementors to use that common functionality as the starting point for their own work, while avoiding large capital investments such as building their own infrastructure and platform. Thus, complementors can now spend their efforts on producing more specialized complements of their product or service, focusing on their core competencies and expertise. The key value proposition for complementors is therefore the elimination of upfront development costs, while benefiting from the common components offered by the platform and while avoiding coordination with other complementors – this is done by the ecosystem orchestrator.[17] Complementors benefit from quick access to an already established market that has relative low barriers to entry.

The alternative would have been to develop an application for a medical device and go to market on their own. The challenge in this scenario is that, irrespective of the performance of their product, the complementors are left with the huge task of marketing that product to healthcare service providers, while trying to convince them of their trustworthiness and sustainability of their business. Thus, digital platform ecosystems offer complementors access to markets that would have been inaccessible to them if they were working in isolation. Indeed, in some cases, without the digital platform ecosystem, complementors may fail to capture their market.

One failed example is Lantern,[18] a mental health startup company that developed digital apps with cognitive behavioral techniques to help mental health patients to deal with stress, anxiety and other mental health issues. Lantern provided these cognitive behavioral techniques directly to patients, but it also employed professional mental healthcare workers as "coaches" to guide patients directly. Lantern's value proposition was based on a direct business-to-consumer business model that failed to gain traction, despite connecting to such employers as Facebook and Intuit. Without an ecosystem orchestrator to establish connections to healthcare providers and employers to scale the business, Lantern was left with the huge task to market its products and services to a wide and growing market for mental healthcare services and to compete with many other different complementors.

Thus, in the same way that an ecosystem orchestrator helps healthcare service providers to more easily search for relevant digital solutions, the orchestrator can help complementors to more easily find relevant customers. In other words, digital platform ecosystems can reduce the search costs for complementors. Transaction and delivery costs are also reduced through the infrastructure of the ecosystem that provides common transaction and exchange mechanisms for all.

As the ecosystem orchestrator coordinates co-opetition between the various ecosystem actors, curating digital services for variety and quality and bringing down costs, patients benefit the most. Patients can gain a wider and more convenient access to higher-quality digital health services at relatively lower costs. More importantly, exactly because of the data-driven nature of these digital solutions across domains of expertise, patients are in a position to benefit from precision medicine, targeted at their individual needs. Digital platform ecosystems can expand the points of care and the service modalities through which patients become empowered and have a choice and control over the way their care is planned and delivered, based on what matters to them and their individual needs. Better informed choices over healthcare services can translate into improved patient outcomes and positive behavioral changes over the management of medical conditions and diseases.

4.2   A Framework for Digital Transformation in Healthcare Ecosystems

The Siemens Healthineers teamplay platform ecosystem offers but one example of how organizations can digitally transform the way they develop and deliver healthcare services. It highlights the co-dependencies between diverse ecosystem actors in relation to their value propositions, while also pointing out the innovation opportunities when combining their unique capabilities and resources in ways not possible if doing so independently from one another. It also highlights how organizations such as Zwanger-Pesiri Radiology can implement and adopt various workflow solutions through the teamplay platform, with support from the team at Siemens Healthineers, but also third-party complementors.

Although digital platform ecosystems like the one orchestrated by Siemens Healthineers look highly successful on the surface with great possibilities for growth and value co-creation, there are a number of challenges involved. These include establishing the right incentives to manage the co-dependencies between ecosystem actors, and on governing the risks of both co-innovation and co-adoption across the ecosystem. This section describes how these risks can be governed so that organizations can leverage the opportunities of an ecosystem approach to digital transformation. Figure 4.1 illustrates the ecosystem digital transformation framework.

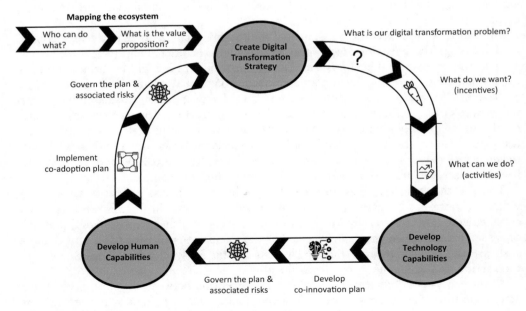

Figure 4.1 The Ecosystem Digital Transformation Framework.

4.2.1 Create the Digital Transformation Strategy: Define Co-dependencies and Establish Incentives

As a first step, when creating their digital transformation strategy, organizations need to define their co-dependencies with other ecosystem actors and establish incentives for motivating collaboration. As discussed in the case of the Siemens Healthineers' platform ecosystem, value propositions need to cut across ecosystem actors such that what is valuable for ecosystem actor A is also valuable for ecosystem actor B. These co-dependencies between ecosystem actors form the "alignment structure" of the ecosystem.[19] Alignment structure refers to the multilateral agreement between ecosystem actors regarding their role and activities such that no actor is in a position to take advantage of other actors or to be better off than them without the ecosystem losing its overall value. What this means is that ecosystem actors need to establish a set of incentives through which they can coordinate their roles and activities. Collectively, all ecosystem actors' roles and activities add up to the reasons why an ecosystem approach to digital transformation is needed and, indeed, why it becomes valuable to all actors. Table 4.2 provides examples of the types of roles and activities that different ecosystem actors can take on, in relation to the digital transformation problem each of them are faced, while also identifying the key incentives that motivate them to participate in the ecosystem.

Device manufacturers and technology providers like Siemens Healthineers have traditionally engaged in transactional business models that relied on one-off sales of hardware and software. For them, the digital transformation problem is developing solutions that allow them to engage in platform business models. These platform business models can enable continuous updates on demand and can generate new digital solutions, while capturing recurring value from users. The primary incentive for device manufacturers and technology providers is thus an opportunity to address this problem, without facing the chicken-and-egg dilemma: without a large user base of healthcare service providers willing to use new digital solutions, no complementor would be incentivized to join the platform and, vice versa, without a good number and variety of digital solutions provided by complementors, no healthcare service provider would be incentivized to join either. Device manufacturers and technology providers are in a perfect position to solve the chicken-and-egg dilemma by building a platform on top of their successful products.[20] For example, Siemens Healthineers has a wide number of very successful products that are already systematically used by healthcare service providers in their routine practices, from MRI to CT scanners and other medical devices. Thus, they essentially already had one side on board. All they had to do was to provide the right incentives for third-party complementors to join the platform (discussed below). A secondary incentive for device manufacturers and technology providers is to mitigate the risks of research and development of new digital solutions, while capturing value from those solutions. In other words, they want to engage in open innovation through third-party complements in order to generate network effects for users, but they want to make sure that any risks are mitigated so as not to impact the first incentive. These risks will be discussed in more detail in the next subsections. To fulfill their role as ecosystem orchestrators, these actors need to provide a modular, scalable technological infrastructure and standard interfaces to deliver digital services on demand, while also providing the necessary governance mechanisms to enable users to interact. Both of these activities are necessary to provide incentives for ecosystem actors.

Table 4.2 The Alignment Structure of a Digital Platform Ecosystem

Ecosystem Actor Role	What Is Our Digital Transformation (DT) Problem?	What Do We Want? (Incentives)	What Can We Do? (Activities)
Ecosystem Orchestrator (e.g., device manufacturers, technology providers)	• Move from transactional to platform business models that have generative value (e.g., one product can spawn new services)	• Primary: address the DT problem without facing the chicken-and-egg dilemma • Secondary: mitigate the risks of research and development of new digital solutions, while capturing value from those solutions	• Provide modular, scalable technological infrastructure and standard interfaces to deliver digital services on demand • Provide technical, financial and behavioral governance mechanisms to enable platform users to interact
Ecosystem Actors (professional users) (e.g., healthcare service providers such as hospitals and diagnostic centers)	• Achieve flexible and scalable technological integration across varied systems and data types	• Primary: address the DT problem at a low cost and without worrying about all the technical complexity involved • Secondary: gain access to value-added services that are curated and trustworthy	• Share data and insights from new technology use • Provide medical domain expertise and knowledge to complement digital solutions
Ecosystem Actors (complementors) (e.g., digital startups such as app developers)	• Avoid large capital investments in technology infrastructure, as well as costs in marketing digital solutions	• Primary: address DT problem, while gaining access to an established market. • Secondary: gain access to data and domain expertise to further improve their digital solutions or even to create yet new services	• Develop specialized digital solutions to address ecosystem actors' needs • Provide technical domain expertise to complement actors' needs

Healthcare service providers like Zwanger-Pesiri Radiology are often faced with the problem of growing their practice, but they do not have the digital maturity to do so, including no human and technological capabilities to integrate all their systems and data types. Flexible and scalable technological integration and interoperability across data types is a common problem across many healthcare service providers and it is usually the key driver behind digital transformation projects. So, the primary incentive for healthcare service providers is to address this problem at a relatively low cost and without worrying about all the technical complexity involved. A secondary incentive is to gain access to value-added services that are curated by the ecosystem orchestrator and that are trustworthy. Healthcare service providers often do not know where to search and which services to select to augment and transform their existing practices. They can identify the big operational and technological challenges they face such as interoperability between systems and data portability and security, but often lack the technical knowledge and expertise to assess the potential impact of new digital solutions to their practices. By joining an ecosystem, all of that is left to the ecosystem orchestrator, who has the capabilities and resources to assess new digital solutions, select the best ones for the ecosystem and implement the right governance mechanisms with which to enable platform users to interact. The potential activities associated with ecosystem actors such as healthcare service providers include sharing data and insights from their use of technology to other ecosystem actors, as well as providing medical domain expertise and knowledge to complement digital solutions.

Digital startups such as software application developers and AI workflow system integrators are faced with the problem of large capital investments in building their own infrastructure and platform, as well as costs in marketing their digital solutions to the market. Many digital startups fail not because their digital solutions are not good enough, but primarily because they are new, unknown and untested in the market with most incumbents ignoring them.[21] Thus, the primary incentive for them is to address their digital transformation problem, while gaining access to an established market. A secondary incentive is to gain access to data and domain expertise that would help these complementors to further improve their digital solutions or even to create yet new services. To fulfill their ecosystem complementor role, these application developers need to engage in activities such as developing specialized digital solutions to address ecosystem actor needs and providing technical domain expertise to complement the medical domain expertise of healthcare service providers.

Certainly, depending on the type of ecosystem actors involved (e.g., payers, pharma and biotech, digital technology providers), the roles, digital transformation problems, incentives and activities will differ. However, for any ecosystem to be formed, there needs to be an alignment structure that is multilaterally agreed by all actors. The next step is to execute the strategy as defined in the alignment structure. In executing the strategy, a number of risks will emerge, including co-innovation and co-adoption risk[22] which are tightly connected to the activities each of the ecosystem actors have agreed to carry out. These risks need to be identified upfront and governed, as discussed in the next two subsections.

4.2.2   *Develop Technology Capabilities: Define A Co-Innovation Plan and Govern Risks*

Once a digital strategy has been developed, while defining the co-dependencies between the various ecosystem actors and establishing incentives such that value is captured by all, the next phase is to develop the technology capabilities that would make the strategy viable. Exactly because of the co-dependencies between ecosystem actors, innovation is a collaborative task with competitive risks. On the one hand, the success of ecosystem actor A's innovation depends on the success of ecosystem actor B's innovation. On the other hand, however, each of these innovations will carry different financial, technical and operational risks. For example, the modular, scalable infrastructure developed by Siemens Healthineers, upon which the teamplay platform is built, carries higher risks than an AI workflow solution developed by a third-party complementor. The level of risk absorbed by each ecosystem actor defines the degree of the value capture they are in a position to claim. This is why, typically, most digital platform ecosystems rest on a higher revenue share capture for the orchestrator than the complementors (e.g., 70/30 percent). Beyond value-capture agreements, however, ecosystem actors have to develop co-innovation plans and govern the risks of those plans so that the ecosystem itself can continue to grow sustainably.

Co-innovation risk is defined as *the "challenge partners face in developing the ability to undertake the new activities that underlie their planned contributions".*[23] Co-innovation risk depends on the *"joint probability" that each ecosystem actor "will be able to satisfy their innovation commitments within a specific time frame".*[24]

Consider the following example. Siemens Healthineers selects a third-party complementor to develop software to analyze cardiac MRI studies. The software is meant to use machine learning algorithms to provide fully automated segmentation of ventricular function, flow and delayed enhancement. The software depends on upgrades of Siemens Healthineers' MRI scanners interfaces, as well as access to healthcare service providers' electronic patient records systems. Each of these three ecosystem actors has to carry out innovations on their systems before the final product is up and running. Let's assume that each of these ecosystem actors has an 80 percent probability that they will be able to deliver their innovations on time to meet the demand of the cardiologists. Together, however, their *"joint probability"* runs down to 51 percent (80 percent × 80 percent × 80 percent).[25] The more ecosystem actors are added to the co-innovation efforts, the more co-innovation risk increases. Complex technologies such as machine learning algorithms may add more complexity and thus lower individual probability of success. This may, in turn, lower the joint probability of the ecosystem actors even more. Certainly, in reality, such probability scores are impossible to calculate precisely. However, what this example shows is that in an ecosystem approach to digital transformation, there are joint risks that cannot be managed by a single actor, nor can one actor's individual probability score significantly lift the joint probability of success for the whole ecosystem. Rather, all actors need to be supported with resources and capabilities to increase their individual probabilities and together raise their joint probability of success.

On digital platform ecosystems, such co-innovation risk can be reduced through the design of the underlying technological architecture.[26] Platform ecosystems benefit from open innovation and scale and scope economies. However, ecosystem orchestrators must coordinate such open innovation to achieve technological integration, while at the same time ensure the autonomy of individual ecosystem actors.[27] In other words, individual ecosystem actors should be autonomous enough to engage in innovation in their vertical and/or horizontal markets. This would ensure the generation of differentiated services and products to serve the needs of yet new ecosystem actors and, thus, contribute to the growth of the ecosystem. At the same time, however, such innovation needs to be coordinated and integrated on the ecosystem in an effort to reduce co-innovation risk. The ecosystem orchestrator needs to build governance mechanisms in the architecture of a digital platform ecosystem to reduce co-innovation risk.

The architecture of a digital platform ecosystem can be decomposed into a set of highly reusable core platform components (e.g., the operating system) that remain relatively stable over time, and a set of complementary components (e.g., the apps provided by third parties) that can vary.[28] The core and complementary components can be integrated through a set of interfaces, which instruct the complementary components on how the platform works, but also how it can be used by these components.[29] Unless the platform core components and the complementary apps can be separated by design, it will become increasingly impossible for them to be developed by independent parties, thus adding to the co-innovation risk. By decomposing these components into separate modules through the architecture, innovation among ecosystem actors can also be separated, thus mitigating risks across them.

Decomposition of the digital platform ecosystem into modular components affects which parts of the ecosystem must be synergistically combined to implement new apps or even to update existing ones. This, in turn, impacts the costs incurred by different ecosystem actors, depending on who is responsible for those new implementations and updates. The more interdependencies between platform core components and complementary apps, as well as between apps themselves, the more difficult integration becomes and the higher the co-innovation risk. This is so because even small changes to one component can have ripple effects on other parts of the ecosystem. This is especially true for apps that are driven by machine learning algorithms that are often tightly coupled to other apps and data resources.[30] The greater the number of components that must be configured in order to successfully change an app, the greater the coordination costs and the co-innovation risk between ecosystem actors. If open innovation by external third parties is to be enabled, these costs and risks must be contained. Architectural differences across platforms can therefore partly explain why co-innovation among ecosystem actors can be significantly different across competing platforms. "Architectural differences can also explain not just the frequency of innovations feasible by app developers but also the types of innovations that do and do not occur in an ecosystem".[31]

Table 4.3 provides a summary of four broad types of platform architectures, while pointing out their trade-offs for the ecosystem orchestrator and the complementors.

Depending on the digital transformation problem being addressed and the key objective of the ecosystem, ecosystem actors will choose a different type of digital platform architecture. Some will want to have more control over the ecosystem, while others will be willing to distribute that control. More control will often be less attractive to complementors, while constraining innovation, whereas less control may offer more open innovation opportunities with the trade-off of fragmentation. Also, it should be noted that some architectures may be orchestrated by a single organization, while others by a consortium of organizations or even a more loosely bounded community of users and complementors, as in the case of loosely coupled architectures with open interfaces and development tools.

First, some companies will adopt a tightly coupled architecture with proprietary interfaces and development tools. For example, Apple has always adopted this first type of architecture for all its products and services, from iMusic to Apple TV and its Apple App Store. Likewise, for its Health App,[34] Apple used a tightly coupled architecture that is centrally controlled by Apple to integrate with all its hardware devices, from iPads and iWatches to Macbook Pros, as well as the various Apple operating systems such as iOS

Table 4.3 Digital Platform Architectures and Their Trade-Offs

Digital Platform Architecture	Trade-offs for the Ecosystem	Who Is This For? Examples
1 Tightly coupled with proprietary interfaces and development tools	• Competitive advantages: This type of architecture provides the highest level of control to the ecosystem orchestrator. Platform core components and complementor apps are centrally integrated with proprietary interfaces and development tools (e.g., Apple Health Records API and Swift[32]) ensuring uniformity in end-user experience. There are also stronger possibilities for achieving higher quality, better security and privacy of health data than in other architectures. The orchestrator is in a better position to align value capture and creation opportunities for platform-native complementors. The platform ecosystem controls for fragmentation and curbs users and complementors from switching to other platforms. • Competitive challenges: Co-innovation risk is high and the ecosystem orchestrator takes full responsibility for managing it. Complementors may be less motivated to participate given the arms-length relationship the platform requires. Innovation is restricted, with high switching costs for complementors.	Organizations that already have one side on board such as the end-users of hardware devices, and that have the market power and technological know-how to orchestrate an ecosystem. Example: *Apple Health platform*
2 Tightly coupled with open interfaces and development tools	• Competitive advantages: The same competitive advantages as above still hold true with the key difference that open interfaces and development tools provide more opportunities for innovation and cross-platform interoperability, without fragmenting the platform. Innovation is enabled given the low switching costs for complementors. There may be innovation spillovers between complementors that benefit other ecosystem actors such as healthcare service providers. • Competitive challenges: Co-innovation risk is still high, because the ecosystem orchestrator now has a more complex system integration task. The coordination costs for the orchestrator, thus, increase. Complementors may be more motivated to participate given that they can develop apps with open development tools (e.g., TensorFlow and CommonHealth SDK[33]). Complementors can, thus, switch to other competing platforms.	Organizations that want to retain some centralized control, while achieving interoperability between multiple sites. Example: *Better Platform* for government and public sector organizations

| 3 Loosely coupled with proprietary interfaces and development tools | • Competitive advantages: Loosely coupled architectures allow individual components to be more independent to one another. The architecture can be vendor agnostic supporting components by multiple different complementors. This type of architecture carries less co-innovation risk than tightly coupled ones: a failed component can be relatively easily removed and replaced by an alternative one. By using proprietary interfaces and development tools, the ecosystem orchestrator achieves distributed integration between platform core and complementary components, without imposing any centralized rules in each ecosystem actor's site.

• Competitive challenges: Coordination costs may rise for the complementors, because, even though the architecture is vendor agnostic, they have to adapt their applications to the architecture's proprietary interfaces. Thus, complementors fall into an arms-length relationship with the ecosystem orchestrator. Even though complementors can develop for other platforms, their innovation on this platform is restricted and has moderate switching costs. | Organizations that, like those in the first type, already have one side on board such as professional users of hardware devices, and also have the market power and technological know-how to orchestrate an ecosystem. Professional users benefit from partnerships with other ecosystem actors, who would not be willing to be locked into a tightly coupled architecture.
Example: *Siemens Healthineers' teamplay platform* |
| 4 Loosely coupled with open interfaces and development tools | • Competitive advantages: The same competitive advantages as above still hold true with the key difference that open interfaces and development tools provide more opportunities for innovation and cross-platform interoperability. This type of architecture offers the highest degree of open innovation opportunities.

• Competitive challenges: The biggest challenge is integration and coordination. The ecosystem orchestrator (usually a community or consortium of organizations) would have a limited ability to enforce common governance rules, which may end up in a "tragedy of the commons", with some complementors free-riding, and fragmenting the platform. The long history of open-source software platforms provides evidence of all the above. Like the first type, this type of architecture carries high co-innovation risk, despite being the most open of all types. | Research organizations and developer communities working closely with ecosystem actors in pilot projects that have small budgets. If successful, such projects will then have to move from prototyping to commercial production with clear governance structures and technical support.
Example: *Open Health Hub's Connected Health platform* |

and MacOS. For Apple, it is important to keep the end-user experience homogeneous and uniform across devices and apps while aiming for higher quality, better security and privacy of health data. This is why Apple requires all apps developed by third parties to use its HealthKit development tool and the Swift programming language, before screening them for approval. Apple has a very strong brand and market position for its hardware devices that allows it to demand from complementors that they only use their proprietary interfaces and tools, while making sure that their apps are tightly coupled with Apple native apps. On the one hand, Apple native complementors (i.e., those that only develop apps for Apple) benefit from all the platform core resources and capabilities provided by Apple. They also benefit from Apple's coordination and governance of the co-innovation risk. On the other hand, for non-native complementors that want to also develop apps for other platforms, this first type of architecture is too constraining with high switching costs. Their efforts and costs will be duplicated if they decide to also develop apps for other platforms. Many small complementors will be completely de-motivated to participate on the platform ecosystem for fear of being locked into Apple's control. This type of architecture may be the best option for a company like Apple, but it will probably not work so well for organizations that do not already have one side on board such as the end-users of hardware devices and that do not have the market power and technological know-how to orchestrate an ecosystem.

The second type of architecture has the same competitive advantages as those discussed above, with the key difference that open interfaces and development tools provide more opportunities for innovation and cross-platform interoperability. Chapter 2 offers an extensive discussion of the different types of APIs used in healthcare and how they interconnect with various health standards such as HL7 and FIHR. The key difference between proprietary and open APIs is that the latter are publicly available and shared under open-source licenses, allowing an ecosystem orchestrator to give a universal access to its complementors. Open APIs can be designed in a variety of different ways,[35] but the main priority of any open API is to be easily accessed and used by as many different complementors as possible. In turn, using proprietary protocols, data formats and developer tools to create open APIs is discouraged, while using open-source technology and open standards is encouraged. Allowing open API on a platform signals to complementors that there is more flexibility in developing components that could integrate with the platform core. However, an open API may still be controlled by the publisher that licenses it – it may be the ecosystem orchestrator or another company. For example, Better Platform[36] provides a tightly coupled, centralized platform architecture for government and public sector organizations, while using open API.[37] This enables innovation for third-party complementors without fragmenting the core platform components. In addition, there may be innovation spillovers between complementors that benefit other ecosystem actors such as healthcare service providers. The key challenge for this type of architecture rests with the ecosystem orchestrator, who now has a more complex system integration task and who is responsible for managing co-innovation risk. In addition, complementors can develop apps for other competing platforms. This type of architecture may work well with organizations that want to retain some centralized control, while achieving interoperability between multiple sites.

Third, unlike tightly coupled architectures, loosely coupled architectures allow individual components to be more independent to one another. Like the Siemens Healthineers teamplay platform, the architecture can be vendor agnostic supporting components by multiple different complementors. The Siemens Healthineers teamplay platform is based on Kubernetes,[38] an open-source architecture developed by Google, making use of proprietary interfaces and development tools provided by Siemens Healthineers such as syngo.via and C-arms.[39] This type of architecture carries less co-innovation risk than tightly coupled ones because a failed component can be relatively easily removed and replaced by an alternative one. By using proprietary interfaces and development tools, the ecosystem orchestrator achieves distributed integration between platform core and complementary components, without imposing any centralized rules in each ecosystem actor's site (e.g., in healthcare service provider's premises). In this way, each ecosystem actor can choose whether to implement a more tightly coupled or a more loosely coupled architecture at their site. The key challenge with this type of architecture is that coordination costs may rise for the ecosystem complementors, because, even though the architecture is vendor agnostic, they have to adapt their applications to the architecture's proprietary interfaces. Thus, complementors fall into an arms-length relationship with the ecosystem orchestrator as in the first type of architecture discussed above. Even though complementors can develop apps for other platforms, their innovation on this platform is restricted and has high switching costs. This type of architecture may work well with organizations that, like those in the first type, already have one side on board such as the end-users of hardware devices and also have the market power and technological know-how to orchestrate an ecosystem. However, the key difference here is that the end-users of hardware devices are professional users that benefit from partnerships with other ecosystem actors, who would not be willing to be locked into a tightly coupled architecture.

The fourth and final type of architecture has the same competitive advantages as those discussed above, with the key difference that open interfaces and development tools provide more opportunities for innovation and cross-platform interoperability. This type of architecture offers the highest range of open innovation opportunities. For example, the Open Health Hub's Connected Health platform[40] enables patients and doctors to securely exchange data and communication between them. The platform is vendor agnostic and device agnostic, thus ensuring maximum interoperability between doctors and patients. Open Health Hub is built using open interfaces and development tools[41] allowing any complementor to participate. The biggest challenge of this type of architecture is integration and coordination. Like other open-source software platforms, the ecosystem orchestrator (usually a community or consortium of organizations) has a limited ability to enforce common governance rules, which may end up in a "tragedy of the commons",[42] with some complementors free-riding and fragmenting the platform. Given that all interfaces and tools are open source, it is relatively easy for competent complementors to reconfigure the code and completely change the functionality of the platform, something which – if done by many complementors – will end up fragmenting the community of doctors and patients that is supported by the platform. Worse yet, complementors may copy the platform's core components to create a completely new platform that directly competes with the host platform while maintaining compatibility with it.[43] The long history of open-source software platforms provides evidence of all the above. Thus, like the first type, this type of architecture carries high co-innovation risk, despite being the most open of all types, since coordinating efforts and ensuring common governance become very difficult. Achieving security will also become very challenging because of the open access to the source code. This type of architecture may work well with research organizations and developer communities working closely with patients and healthcare service providers in pilot projects that have small budgets. If successful, such projects will then have to move from prototyping to commercial production with clear governance structures and technical support. This move usually means becoming integrated into one of the architecture types discussed above.

The four types of platform architectures discussed above are quite broad in scope. Many ecosystems will implement variations of these architectures, with some components being tightly coupled and others being loosely coupled. The key objective of this discussion is not to point out which architecture is best nor to provide a complete technical specification of how various components should interact. Rather, the key objective is to highlight the trade-offs involved for different ecosystem actors, as they exchange resources and capabilities to develop new digital technologies. Depending on the choice of platform architecture, there will be different competitive advantages, as well as challenges in governing co-innovation risk.

4.2.3   Develop Human Capabilities: Implement A Co-Adoption Plan and Govern Risks

The next phase is to develop human capabilities within each organization participating in the ecosystem for transitioning their work to the new digital technologies. Once again, exactly because of the co-dependencies between ecosystem actors, the implementation and adoption of new digital technologies is a collaborative task. Thus, whereas previous approaches have placed emphasis on the individual user acceptance of technology and adoption by groups within single organizations,[44] the ecosystem approach places emphasis on implementation and adoption across organizational boundaries. Certainly, like earlier approaches, attention must still be paid on individual users of technology to assess improvements in productivity and task performance within each participating organization. However, in an ecosystem approach, ecosystem actors have to coordinate their efforts to also govern co-adoption risk.

Co-adoption risk is defined as *the extent to which ecosystem actors adopt the new technologies to capture the value-in-use of their co-innovation plan.* Co-adoption risk will vary depending on the digital maturity of each actor regarding their human capabilities. The digital maturity of ecosystem actors will affect their capability to enforce a set of collective action rules that balance the benefits and costs of the new technologies.

Organizations with low digital maturity will face the most challenges when it comes to governing co-adoption risk. Unless these organizations quickly transform to catch up with new digital initiatives across the ecosystem, they will be constantly disrupted, something which may eventually lead to their collapse. Healthcare service providers such as public sector hospitals who are troubled by shortages in public sector funding and have limited capacity to train their staff in the use of new technologies usually exhibit low digital maturity.[45] Most healthcare service providers struggle to meet existing patient needs while undergoing digital transformation, with staff – from admin to clinical staff – having to work overtime to meet technology go-live and upgrades. Indeed, the upfront adoption costs of digital transformation for healthcare service providers often exceed the benefits, and this is why many providers keep postponing change projects, while healthcare staff keep resisting technology.[46] In such cases, digital transformation teams will have to first and foremost develop plans for upskilling staff and upgrading technology to meet the needs of individual organizations prior to participating in an ecosystem. Individual organizations will have to develop a coherent company-wide policy and program of hiring and training staff in digital skills relevant to their respective specializations and functional units. All executive leaders will have to be trained with a digital competency and a digital-first mindset to understand how digital technologies can transform their units. In addition, individual organizations will have to develop a technology architecture and governance model that supports both core centralized systems and other digital technologies across functional units, while offering a coherent, end-to-end, fully digitized experience for staff and customers as discussed in Chapter 3.

As these healthcare service providers become more digitally mature, they will begin to have higher demands from the ecosystem. For example, a hospital may demand from Siemens Healthineers to assign new technical teams to take on the task of integrating new technologies from third-party complementors on existing medical devices such as MRI scanners. These teams comprising internal hospital staff and technical staff from Siemens Healthineers will work closely with the complementors to assess the new components, test them off the teamplay platform and pilot them in specific units in the hospital. They will be in a position to then prepare training and implementation plans for healthcare and administrative staff, while the third-party complementors would be in a position to offer technical support.

Large healthcare service providers with a wealth of digital resources and capabilities may even start to compete with complementors by developing their own complements and making them available on the digital platform. In the English NHS, there is a lot of duplication of services, especially support services such as portering, security, receipt and distribution, telecoms and non-emergency patient transport. Each NHS Hospital contracts with different suppliers for these services. A great outlier is Barts Health NHS Trust that, on 1 May 2023, insourced a contract from SERCO after years of insufficient services and cashflow problems.[47] Barts Health NHS Trust is one of the biggest healthcare providers in the English NHS, with four hospitals, including one teaching hospital and serving 2.5 million patients. By insourcing these support services, Barts Health NHS Trust could eventually become a shared services center for other smaller hospitals. This transition is supported by a third party, Synbiotix Solutions Limited,[48] that provided the digital solution for the shared services. Thus, unlike co-innovation risk that can largely be governed through the technology architecture of the platform ecosystem, co-adoption risk requires behavioral governance mechanisms that help address collective action problems.

Similarly, digitally mature complementors may start to compete with other less mature complementors and even the ecosystem orchestrators themselves. The ecosystem orchestrator needs to work closely with all ecosystem actors to develop a co-adoption plan that will take into consideration the benefit-to-cost ratio for each actor. If one set of actors is left to carry the cost of digital transformation alone, while others benefit, the collective value proposition of the ecosystem may never be realized. The ecosystem orchestrator needs to discourage opportunistic behavior, while maximizing value creation at different levels of digital maturity.

Table 4.4 provides a summary of the potential collective action problems that may arise between ecosystem actors at different levels of digital maturity, while also highlighting the relevant governance mechanisms that could help address those problems.

Effective governance is achieved through incentive alignment and authority allocation (i.e., control).[49] Authority allocation can be defined in relation to various decisions rights ranging from how the platform core and the modular components function and interact with one another through various interfaces.[50] Incentive alignment involves monetary and non-monetary rewards such as privileges or reputation. Incentive alignment occurs when the platform's functionality induces use consistent with the design objective.[51]

Table 4.4 Collective Action Problems and Governance Mechanisms

Digital Maturity of Ecosystem Actors	Potential Collective Action Problems	Governance Mechanisms
Low	1. Coordination problems between technical teams of diverse ecosystem actors (e.g., technical issues – including use of standards and interfaces, but also technical support – emerging during pilot, go-live and full implementation of the digital platform and of complementary apps) 2. Concerns over security compliance, ethics and privacy of data 3. Competition over pricing of digital products and services 4. Resistance by staff (e.g., doctors) due to conflicts with workload, lack of skills and non-acceptance of the technology, perceived lack of engagement, inconsistency with organizational values and other related issues	1. Design architectural control and access to core and peripheral components (see Table 4.3 for varied configurations) 2. Allocate and enforce decision rights over data access, storage and processing 3. Allocate and enforce pricing rights (e.g., revenue share, transaction fees, subscription). Specify incentives (e.g., rewards based on performance) 4. Provide training and showcase benefits of the technology (e.g., quality of care, efficiency of clinical practices, productivity gains). Ensure the professional autonomy of staff and establish links to organizational values
Medium	5. Misalignments between upgrades to core platform components and complementary apps (e.g., impacting decision and pricing rights) 6. Platform leakage (e.g., users and complementors interact off the platform) 7. Information asymmetries between ecosystem actors	5. Implement gatekeeping (e.g., ensure compliance to architectural design and rights allocation) 6. Avoid escalating transaction fees. Offer incentives in the form of value-added services (e.g., performance metrics). Make services tightly coupled to core platform components 7. Implement decision-making rights for handling data in different locations
High	8. Competitive frictions • Complementors can develop apps for competing platforms • Enveloping or crowding out of complementary apps by large complementors (e.g., launching similar apps or adding similar features on existing apps) • Self-preferencing or discrimination of apps • Free-riding by some complementors (e.g., capitalize on innovations by others, use resources without contributions) 9. Neglecting low value users by some complementors and focusing only on high value users. Decreasing quality and performance of services offered because of price competition 10. Manipulating ratings and reviews by ecosystem actors	8. Establish contractual agreements with exclusivity clauses (e.g., no development for competing platforms or only after a specific time has lapsed). Add switching costs in the form of proprietary interfaces and standards. Implement graduated sanctions depending on impact of anti-competitive practices and opportunistic behavior 9. Exercise performance control and provide incentives (e.g., pecuniary and promotional rewards) based on market performance and user ratings and reviews. Curate list of complementors based on performance, uniqueness of complements and value creation opportunities 10. Implement machine learning tools to better detect rating and review manipulations

As discussed already in the previous section, both of these governance mechanisms can be implemented in the design of the technological architecture of digital platform ecosystems. However, these need to be enforced with behavioral mechanisms, which will vary at different levels of digital maturity. In addition, depending on the key objective of the ecosystem and its associated platform architecture, these governance mechanisms may need to be enforced by a single ecosystem orchestrator or a consortium of organizations.

First, organizations that undergo digital transformation through an ecosystem approach for the first time will exhibit low digital maturity, even if they have previously implemented digital technologies in their organization. One of the key collective action problems they will be faced with is that of coordinating with other ecosystem actors on the technical aspects of their digital transformation. For example, technical teams from Siemens Healthineers will have to coordinate with the technical teams of healthcare service providers and even with third-party complementors to resolve such issues as migrating legacy technology and data to the teamplay platform and making sure that common standards and interfaces are used by all. Technical support by Siemens Healthineers and third-party complementors will also have to be provided during pilot, go-live and full implementation of the teamplay platform, as well as any complementary apps. Such technical coordination can be achieved by designing control mechanisms in the technological architecture of the platform. These technical control mechanisms can define access to core and peripheral components, while also specifying what kind of standards and interfaces will be used to achieve integration and interoperability between components, including how complementors can develop and submit apps to be added onto the platform (e.g., development environments, SDK and API). Depending on the digital transformation problem and key objective of the ecosystem, different control mechanisms can be implemented, as summarized in Table 4.3.

Second, organizations with low digital maturity will also have concerns about the ways by which the new digital technologies are compliant to existing security rules and protocols, whether they account for ethical policies and whether they protect the privacy of patient data. As discussed in Chapter 2, even though ecosystem orchestrators with cloud-based digital platforms already embed compliance to such regulations as HIPAA in the USA and GDPR in Europe in their technologies, data practices may vary between and across ecosystem actors. Orchestrators should define and enforce a set of decision rights on how data are accessed, stored and processed by each ecosystem actor.[52] Roles such as data custodians (e.g., healthcare service providers) and data consumers (e.g., app developers) could help define the decision rights of each actor, while the orchestrator ensures that technical and behavioral mechanisms of security and privacy compliance are enforced (e.g., authenticating users, anonymizing data, providing opt-out choices).

Third, organizations participating in a platform ecosystem may have concerns over their ability to set prices for their digital products and services, while competing with others in the same market. On the one hand, competition brings down prices for users (e.g., healthcare service providers) and, by extension, patients too. But, on the other hand, if there is too much competition on prices, organizations become disincentivized to join a platform ecosystem. The ecosystem orchestrator may allocate and enforce pricing rights for each type of ecosystem actor based on the key objectives of the ecosystem. For example, in the case of Apple Health, complementors enter a revenue share agreement with Apple, starting with 70/30 percent and moving to 85/15 percent if the apps manage to secure annual subscriptions from end-users. In this case, the complementors can set the price for their apps and services, but their revenues will be capped at 70 percent or

85 percent depending on subscriptions. Other platforms may charge institutional users such as hospitals a recurring subscription fee to access a complementary app, or charge both hospitals and complementors a transaction fee for allowing them to interact on the platform for additional services (e.g., an analysis report), depending on how the ecosystem is set up. In the case of subscription fees, all products and services are bundled at a single price. This works well when there is large variance in users' willingness-to-pay across the various products and services offered on the platform.[53] However, subscription pricing could reduce the ability to charge more to users that consume more products and services, while also killing innovation by complementors who may produce specialized complements.[54] This is where providing additional incentives to reward complementors for superior performance or for "superstar" complements could help alleviate some of the aforementioned concerns. Once again, these types of governance mechanisms may be relevant for some ecosystems but not for others.

Fourth, like more conventional approaches to digital transformation, platform ecosystems may be faced with resistance by staff (e.g., clinicians) due to conflicts with workload, lack of skills and non-acceptance of the technology, perceived lack of engagement, inconsistency with organizational values and other related issues. Although this is not a collective action problem directly associated with digital platform ecosystems, it can indirectly impact the formation and growth of a platform ecosystem. Previous research on the implementation of new technologies in healthcare organizations has shown that dealing with staff resistance requires providing training and showcasing the benefits that the technology can provide in relation to the quality of care, efficiency of clinical practices and associated productivity gains.[55] In addition, the same research has shown that staff, especially doctors and nurses, need to be assured that their professional autonomy will not be affected by the new technology and that organizational values are not overlooked.[56] For example, radiologists using the AI-Rad Companion product deployed via the Siemens Healthineers teamplay platform need to be assured that their decision-making authority is not compromised. Such workflow solutions should not interfere with healthcare professionals' clinical practices nor change their professional status vis-à-vis their patients. Organizational values regarding medical accountability, ethics and transparency should be supported through the technology. There is a long list of studies stressing the importance of accounting for all the above to mitigate resistance by staff and successfully transition to new technologies.[57]

As organizations become more digitally mature, a number of other collective action problems may emerge. During upgrades to core and complementary components, new tensions and misalignments may emerge between ecosystem actors. Complementors may seek to implement new features in their applications that allow more data parameters to be captured, that permit "sideloading"[58] of affiliated applications to the platform or that enable purchases to be made off the platform. All these problems were faced by Apple on its App Store, when various developers sought to bypass Apple's governance mechanisms with a significant impact on existing decision and pricing rights.[59] To address these problems, the ecosystem orchestrator can implement gatekeeping, that is, screening out apps that do not comply to existing architectural design and rights allocation.[60] Such screening can be done using both machine learning algorithms and human auditing of apps submitted to a platform's marketplace.

Sixth, another collective action problem that may emerge as organizations become more digitally mature is platform leakage. Platform leakage, that is, users and complementors interacting off the platform, usually takes place after different ecosystem actors meet and decide to enter a bilateral agreement to continue to interact while avoiding platform fees.[61] Platform leakage may also occur because ecosystem actors do not see any value in interacting with more than one other actor who assumingly offers all services they want, or because the platform itself offers no added value to the transactions (e.g., there are no technological benefits). Stagnacy in co-innovation and the generation of new value creation opportunities may also push actors to pivot to bilateral agreements. So, fees, variation in the community of service providers and technological benefits but also stagnancy in co-innovation can all add to platform leakage.

Ecosystem orchestrators can govern the risks of this problem by avoiding escalating transaction fees or even considering a completely different pricing model, as discussed above. The orchestrator may also consider making services more tightly coupled to core platform components such that all transactions – from searching, selecting and paying for services – take place through the platform and not through third-party apps. The more integrated core components are with third-party complements, the less likely ecosystem actors would want to leave the platform because by leaving they would lose access to a wider set of services that could be expensive to access elsewhere. In fact, this is the key reason why Apple wants everything to be centrally integrated on their platform; it wants to control the user experience while mitigating the risk of platform leakage. Finally, the orchestrator may offer incentives in the form of value-added services such as metrics on app performance and related services that would make it more attractive for ecosystem actors to stay on the platform.

Another problem that may occur has to do with information asymmetries between ecosystem actors. Although platform ecosystems may lower information costs for users because they centralize information about available services and products and provide better matching between them, some actors, including the orchestrator, may hold exclusive control over some type of information and data. This may result in a number of information market failures[62] that may benefit some actors, while hurting others. For example, hospitals may only be provided with targeted information about specific complementors, when, in fact, alternative complementors may better serve their needs. Orchestrators may do this to mitigate the risk of platform leakage as discussed above, but, in the process, they may compromise the efficiency of the platform's marketplace. On the other hand, full information disclosure about all products and services, including access to all user data, may weaken incentives for complementors and compromise the protection of data privacy. A solution to narrow the gap between the private and collective welfare value of data within platform ecosystems is to implement decision-making rights over data in relation to their origin location.[63] Instead of allowing transfers of data between ecosystem actors – as proposed in the EU's GDPR "data portability right" – such decision-making rights allow third parties to bring their algorithms on the platform and access data that original data holders (e.g., hospitals) hold at their premises. The data never leaves the data holders' premises, and exclusive control still remains with them. However, third parties can access these data remotely, "in the context of other products and other consumers" while they "propose competing offers".[64] This approach prevents data leakage and reinforces data privacy and security, but would be more relevant in more mature platform ecosystems, with ecosystem actors having developed an understanding of how data can be used and what algorithms could be deployed. Chapter 6 discusses how such data access rights can be applied in the context of Lifebit. AI's unique federated computation analysis platform.[65]

As organizations and the digital platform ecosystem achieve high digital maturity, a number of competitive frictions will start to emerge. The first such friction is between the orchestrator and the complementors who may start to develop apps for other platforms. It is in the complementors' best interest to develop applications for multiple platforms because that would increase their exposure to a wider user base. As discussed in the previous section, the ecosystem orchestrator can make it very difficult for complementors to develop apps for competing platforms by enforcing integration with proprietary standards and interfaces, as well as tightly coupling complementary components to core platform components. At the same time, depending on the key objectives of the ecosystem, the orchestrator (e.g., a national payer) may not want to restrict development for other platforms, at least not entirely. The orchestrator may establish contractual agreements with exclusivity clauses, whereby such development is only allowed after certain conditions have been met or only after a specific time has lapsed to allow the platform ecosystem to grow. Although value capture will increase if no development to competing platforms is allowed, it will also have the adverse effect of reducing innovation spillovers. This is a trade-off that needs to be governed in the context of the key value propositions of the ecosystem.

Other competitive frictions include enveloping or crowding out of complementary apps by large complementors (e.g., launching similar apps or offering similar features as other apps); self-preferencing or discriminating against certain apps; and free-riding by some complementors. Interestingly, some of these frictions may be caused by the orchestrator, signaling a Red Queen race between complementors and further inducing innovation spillovers between them.[66] However, it may also be caused by large complementors and even other large ecosystem actors (e.g., large hospitals) who acquire teams of complementors and become aggregators of complements themselves.[67] In large platform ecosystems, such aggregation may add value via economies of scope and scale. However, in smaller ecosystems, such aggregation may kill competition altogether (although it may be beneficial for smaller complementors who want to develop apps for multiple platforms). In these cases, the orchestrator may need to implement graduated sanctions depending on the impact of anti-competitive practices and opportunistic behavior of different ecosystem actors. Such sanctions may include financial penalties and even removal from the platform.

Further, over time, some complements that were originally introduced as add-ons to the core technology architecture, serving the needs of only a select few users, may become core technology: all or the majority of users demand the complement as a core service of the digital platform. In that case, the ecosystem orchestrator may decide to acquire the complement or to develop a native component that has the same features as the original complement. This is a case of enveloping. However, to avoid friction, the ecosystem orchestrator may offer an exit strategy for the complementor that (a) allows the complementor to make a return on their investment within a reasonable timeframe while allowing them to migrate into new development efforts and (b) sends the signal to other complementors that innovation is valued on the platform ecosystem. These two points are critical for the sustainability of the ecosystem.

The aforementioned competitive frictions, if left unchecked, may reduce the incentives for novel, high-quality complements and for high-quality user support. Some (especially smaller complementors) may end up locked into a platform where they confront very powerful competitors for their products. This co-opetition tension complementors face can lengthen their time to market by pushing them to choose launch dates far removed from those of other platform products. These value-capture problems can ultimately make the platform unattractive[68] for some complementors where a greater proportion of low-quality complements are on offer. Complementors are more likely to launch their innovative complements on new, less crowded platforms, even if these platforms have a smaller installed user base. In these cases, the orchestrator needs to exercise performance control and provide incentives (e.g., pecuniary and promotional rewards) based on market performance and user ratings and reviews. The orchestrator may decide to curate the list of complementors on the platform based on their performance, uniqueness of complements and value creation opportunities.

Finally, the platform ecosystem may suffer from another set of anti-competitive tactics employed by ecosystem actors in relation to false marketing by means of manipulation of ratings and reviews.[69] The presence of difficult to detect fake reviews may misguide users to make suboptimal choices and may also lead to a general mistrust of reviews, both of which can lead to information market failures, as discussed earlier. Although this is a problem primarily found in e-commerce, restaurant and travel platforms, it has also impacted healthcare platforms with fake patient reviews.[70] In recent years, a number of machine learning tools have been developed[71] to better detect rating and review manipulations on different platform ecosystems.

The aforementioned collective action problems are examples of problems a digital platform ecosystem may face once it is implemented and co-adopted by all ecosystem actors. Evidently, these collective action problems will vary depending on the level of digital maturity of ecosystem actors, as well as the platform ecosystem itself. Most importantly, however, these collective action problems point at the distinct governance mechanisms an ecosystem orchestrator needs to implement to coordinate the various ecosystem actors. These governance mechanisms go beyond coordinating the adoption of technology in a single organization, focusing instead on the governance of co-adoption risks.

4.3 The Patients' Perspective

The previous sections have focused primarily on digital transformation from the perspective of ecosystem actors such as technology providers, hospitals and third-party application developers. However, these healthcare ecosystems are very much defined by the needs of different patients and their associated healthcare journeys. Healthcare ecosystems are patient centered, whether directly supporting patient-to-doctor interactions or indirectly contributing to different processes in the healthcare delivery cycle.

Around the world, many patients are becoming more empowered to make healthcare decisions. Increased internet access and the growing use of digital and wearable devices have fundamentally altered the information available to patients, who now expect to be involved when and how treatment choices are made. Patients today have a much better understanding of actionable, lifestyle prescriptions that can reduce the risk of disease and demand more and better knowledge about genetic risks. The shift toward personalized or precision medicine has expanded the list of care points through which patients become empowered and have a choice and control over the way their care is planned and delivered.

This has led to the development of platform ecosystems that leverage not only the capabilities and resources of third-party complementors, but also those of the patients themselves, their families and communities in delivering better outcomes and experiences. These include PatientsLikeMe (recently acquired by UnitedHealth Group[72]),

HealthUnlocked (recently acquired by CorEvitas[73]) and The Mighty that offer online tools for patients to share knowledge about their medical condition with others who have the same medical condition. Patients have an opportunity to monitor their symptoms, understand the treatments that they have available to them and self-manage their medical condition in a way that has not been available to them before. Patient communities on these platforms support one another and teach each other about both the medical aspects of their conditions, but also how to live with different conditions such as breast cancer or epilepsy. While evidence about how community participation shapes medical outcomes is limited, these online communities appear to positively affect members psychologically.[74] Participation heightens levels of emotional well-being and contributes to overall personal empowerment, which in some cases translates into improved decision-making and positive behavioral changes.[75]

Such platform ecosystems provide digital tools for patients to add and review structured health information. On PatientsLikeMe, for example, data entered by patients are compiled and presented as a health history profile and shared within the platform.[76] At the top of each profile is a primary outcomes chart. Depending on the community, the chart displays functional-level results over time. In the case of amyotrophic lateral sclerosis, for example, the primary chart is a line graph of the individual's functional level over time, superimposed against a backdrop of population-level data. Below the primary outcome chart are modified Gantt charts displaying the treatments taken and symptoms experienced.[77] The profile is available for personal use and to be browsed and critiqued by other members.

Patient-centered digital platform ecosystems can aggregate data from all individuals in the community to create summaries of treatments and symptoms for common conditions. Each treatment report shows the dosages, scheduling, indications, perceived efficacy and side effects experienced. Symptom reports list the prevalence and severity of the symptoms experienced and each element in these reports is hyperlinked to related items of interest. In addition, using search and browsing tools, members can locate other patients in similar circumstances and with shared medical experiences. Members can find others by demographic variables, treatment experiences and symptom histories and discuss the profiles and reports, as well as general health concerns, through private messages and comments they post on one another's profiles.

As more ecosystem actors demand data-driven, patient-centered solutions, these digital platform ecosystems may play a new role in the shifting patient–provider relationship. For example, The Mighty provides data analytics capabilities and anonymized patient data on conditions and comorbidities, as well as behavioral data to pharma companies, clinical teams and payers and providers via a cloud platform. Such capabilities and data resources are extremely valuable to these ecosystem actors because they enable them to improve outcomes for their patients and decrease the costs of delivering high-quality services.[78]

Moreover, these patient-centered solutions feed into and leverage new technologies such as whole genome sequencing. Whole genome sequencing companies like Illumina act as the platform ecosystem orchestrators servicing healthcare providers and patients, while building on the complementary services of third parties. For example, using Illumina's platform ecosystem, the Global Genomics Group led a global project across 48 participating clinical sites in nine countries and involving nearly 8,000 patients to identify the specific genotypes of hereditary cardiovascular disease.[79] By identifying those genotypes, they were then able to do whole genome sequencing and target the disease. This has a huge impact on how doctors look at the individual profiles of patients to prescribe therapies that will work not in a population but for specific patients.

As these examples show, there is a wide variety of healthcare ecosystems leveraging the power of digital platforms and generating innovative solutions for improved patient outcomes. Patients will never see the complexity behind these innovative solutions. However, they demand these solutions, and it is exactly such demand that is driving digital transformation across healthcare ecosystems. Ecosystem actors need to get digital transformation right by establishing the appropriate incentives to manage the co-dependencies between them, and by governing the risks of both co-innovation and co-adoption.

Notes

1 https://www.doccla.com/
2 Guk, K., Han, G., Lim, J., Jeong, K., Kang, T., Lim, E.K. and Jung, J., 2019. Evolution of wearable devices with real-time disease monitoring for personalized healthcare. *Nanomaterials*, 9(6), p. 813; Kim, J., Campbell, A.S., de Ávila, B.E.F. and Wang, J., 2019. Wearable biosensors for healthcare monitoring. *Nature Biotechnology*, 37(4), pp. 389–406; Piwek, L., Ellis, D.A., Andrews, S. and Joinson, A., 2016. The rise of consumer health wearables: promises and barriers. *PLoS Medicine*, 13(2), p. e1001953.
3 https://www.ft.com/partnercontent/ping-an-insurance/underwriting-chinas-health-transformation.html
4 https://www.pharmaceutical-technology.com/features/amazon-pharmacy-disruption-healthcare/
5 Joglekar, N., Parker, G. and Srai, J.S., 2020. Winning the race for survival: how advanced manufacturing technologies are driving business-model innovation. *World Economic Forum*. https://www3.weforum.org/docs/WEF_Winning_The_Race_For_Survival_2020.pdf
6 Jacobides, M.G., Cennamo, C. and Gawer, A., 2018. Towards a theory of ecosystems. *Strategic Management Journal*, 39(8), pp. 2255–2276.
7 https://www.siemens-healthineers.com/en-uk/digital-health-solutions/teamplay-digital-health-platform/teamplay-digital-health-platform-as-a-service
8 https://www.siemens-healthineers.com/digital-health-solutions/digital-solutions-overview/clinical-decision-support/ai-rad-companion
9 MedTech Industry Leverages Platform as a Service (PaaS) to Overcome Hurdles, Capitalize on Big Data and Truly Embrace Digital Transformation. *White Paper*. Frost & Sullivan for Siemens Healthineers. https://cdn0.scrvt.com/39b415fb07de4d9656c7b516d8e2d907/17096e0c6eaa3521/87fa86fde3cc/FS_WP_Siemens_Healthineers_teamplay-PaaS.pdf
10 https://marketplace.teamplay.siemens.com/apps
11 Parker, G.G., Van Alstyne, M.W., and Choudary, S.P., 2016. *Platform Revolution: How Networked Markets Are Transforming the Economy and How to Make Them Work for You*. New York: W. W. Norton; Constantinides, P., Henfridsson, O. and Parker, G.G., 2018. Platforms and infrastructures in the digital age. *Information Systems Research*, 29(2), pp. 381–400.
12 Tiwana, A., 2013. *Platform Ecosystems: Aligning Architecture, Governance, and Strategy*. Newnes, Boston, USA.
13 https://marketplace.teamplay.siemens.com/app/detail/AMRA-Researcher
14 Parker G.G., Van Alstyne M.W. and Choudary S.P., 2016. *Platform Revolution: How Networked Markets Are Transforming the Economy and How to Make Them Work for You*. New York: W. W. Norton.
15 Fürstenau, D., Klein, S., Vogel, A. and Auschra, C., 2021. Multi-sided platform and data-driven care research: A longitudinal case study on business model innovation for improving care in complex neurological diseases. *Electronic Markets*, 31, pp. 811–828.
16 Nalebuff, B. J., Brandenburger, A. and Maulana, A. 1996. *Co-opetition*. London: Harper Collins Business; Bengtsson, M. and Kock, S., 2000. "Coopetition" in business networks—to cooperate and compete simultaneously. *Industrial Marketing Management*, 29(5), pp. 411–426; Gnyawali, D.R. and Park, B.J.R., 2011. Co-opetition between giants: collaboration with competitors for technological innovation. *Research Policy*, 40(5), pp. 650–663; Cozzolino, A., Corbo, L. and

Aversa, P., 2021. Digital platform-based ecosystems: the evolution of collaboration and competition between incumbent producers and entrant platforms. *Journal of Business Research*, 126, pp. 385–400.

17 Tiwana, A., 2013. *Platform Ecosystems: Aligning Architecture, Governance, and Strategy.* Newnes.

18 See https://techcrunch.com/2018/07/24/mental-health-startup-lantern-winds-down-its-customer-operations/

19 Adner, R., 2017. Ecosystem as structure: an actionable construct for strategy. *Journal of Management*, 43(1), pp. 39–58.

20 Parker G.G., Van Alstyne M.W., Choudary S.P., 2016. *Platform Revolution: How Networked Markets Are Transforming the Economy and How to Make Them Work for You.* New York: W. W. Norton; also read the very insightful blog by Andrei Hagiu and Julian Wright on how the chicken-and-egg problem can be solved https://platformchronicles.substack.com/p/the-chicken-and-egg-problem-of-marketplaces

21 Christensen, C., 1997. *The Innovator's Dilemma.* Harvard Business School Press, Boston, USA.

22 Adner, R., 2017. Ecosystem as structure: an actionable construct for strategy. *Journal of Management*, 43(1), pp. 39–58; Adner, R., 2012. *The Wide Lens: A New Strategy for Innovation.* Penguin, London UK.

23 Adner, R., 2017. Ecosystem as structure: an actionable construct for strategy. *Journal of Management*, 43(1), p. 48.

24 Adner, R., 2012. *The Wide Lens: A New Strategy for Innovation.* Penguin, London UK. p. 46.

25 Adner, R., 2012. *The Wide Lens: A New Strategy for Innovation.* Penguin, London UK.

26 Tiwana, A., 2013. *Platform Ecosystems: Aligning Architecture, Governance, and Strategy.* Newnes; Yoo, Y., Henfridsson, O., & Lyytinen, K., 2010. The new organizing logic of digital innovation: an agenda for information systems research. *Information Systems Research*, 21(4), pp. 724–735.

27 Fürstenau, D., Auschra, C., Klein, S. and Gersch, M., 2019. A process perspective on platform design and management: evidence from a digital platform in health care. *Electronic Markets*, 29, pp. 581–596.

28 Baldwin, C.Y. and Woodard, C.J., 2009. The architecture of platforms: a unified view. *Platforms, Markets and Innovation*, 32, pp. 19–44.

29 Parnas, D.L., Clements, P.C. and Weiss, D.M., 1985. The modular structure of complex systems. *IEEE Transactions on Software Engineering*, 11 (3), pp. 259–266.

30 Sculley, D., Holt, G., Golovin, D., Davydov, E., Phillips, T., Ebner, D., Chaudhary, V., Young, M., Crespo, J.F. and Dennison, D., 2015. Hidden technical debt in machine learning systems. *Advances in Neural Information Processing Systems*, 28, pp. 2503–2511.

31 Tiwana, A., 2013. *Platform Ecosystems: Aligning Architecture, Governance, and Strategy.* Newnes.

32 See https://www.apple.com/healthcare/health-records/ and https://developer.apple.com/documentation/healthkit/samples/accessing_health_records/

33 See for example https://blog.tensorflow.org/2020/04/ai-for-medicine-specialization-featuring-tensorflow.html and https://www.commonhealth.org/developers

34 https://www.apple.com/ios/health/

35 See for example a list of different open API developed on GitHub https://github.com/search?q=health+api

36 https://platform.better.care/

37 See a description of Better's OpenEHR API https://blog.better.care/better-releases-its-proprietary-openehr-resources-as-open-source released on GitHub https://github.com/better-care

38 https://www.aquasec.com/cloud-native-academy/kubernetes-101/kubernetes-architecture/

39 https://www.siemens-healthineers.com/digital-health-solutions/digital-technologies/digital-marketplace-become-a-partner

40 https://www.openhealthhub.com/hub/connected-health/

41 https://developer.openhealthhub.com/#introduction

42 Hardin, G., 1968. The tragedy of the commons: the population problem has no technical solution; it requires a fundamental extension in morality. *Science*, 162(3859), pp. 1243–1248. See how the tragedy of the commons apply to technologies in healthcare in Constantinides, P., 2012. *Perspectives and Implications for the Development of Information Infrastructures.*

IGI Global, Hershey, USA; Constantinides, P. and Barrett, M., 2015. Information infrastructure development and governance as collective action. *Information Systems Research*, 26(1), pp. 40–56. Also see how it applies to platform ecosystems in Cennamo, C. and Santaló, J., 2019. Generativity tension and value creation in platform ecosystems. *Organization Science*, 30(3), pp. 617–641; O'Mahony, S. and Karp, R., 2020. From proprietary to collective governance: how do platform participation strategies evolve?. *Strategic Management Journal*, 43(3), pp. 530–562.

43 Karhu, K., Gustafsson, R. and Lyytinen, K., 2018. Exploiting and defending open digital platforms with boundary resources: Android's five platform forks. *Information Systems Research*, 29(2), pp. 479–497.

44 For example, see the Technology Acceptance Model (TAM), which is based on the theory of planned behavior (TPB), Venkatesh, V., Davis, F.D. and Morris, M.G., 2007. Dead or alive? The development, trajectory and future of technology adoption research. *Journal of the Association for Information Systems*, 8(4), 268–286; Venkatesh, V., Morris, M.G., Davis, G.B., & Davis, F.D. (2003). User acceptance of information technology: toward a unified view. *MIS Quarterly*, 27(3), 425–478; Sarker, S., & Valacich, J.S. (2010). An alternative to methodological individualism: a non-reductionist approach to studying technology adoption by groups. *MIS Quarterly*, 34(4), 779–808; Sarker, S., Valacich, J.S. and Sarker, S. (2005). Technology adoption by groups: a valence perspective. *Journal of the Association for Information Systems*, 6(2), 37–71.

45 Eden, R., Jones, A.B., Casey, V. and Draheim, M., 2019. Digital transformation requires workforce transformation. *MIS Quarterly Executive*, 18(1), p. 4.

46 Agarwal, R., Gao, G., DesRoches, C. and Jha, A.K., 2010. Research commentary—the digital transformation of healthcare: current status and the road ahead. *Information Systems Research*, 21(4), pp. 796–809.

47 https://www.bartshealth.nhs.uk/news/latest-news-serco-to-pull-out-of-barts-health-facilities-management-in-2023-11969

48 https://www.synbiotix.com/

49 Ostrom, E., 1990. *Governing the Commons*. Cambridge, UK: Cambridge University Press; Williamson, O.E., 1996. *The Mechanisms of Governance*. New York, NY: Oxford University Press.

50 Tiwana, A., 2013. *Platform Ecosystems: Aligning Architecture, Governance, and Strategy*. Newnes.

51 Ba, S., Stallaert, J. and Whinston, A.B. (2001). Research commentary: introducing a third dimension in information systems design – the case for incentive alignment. *Information Systems Research*, 12(3), 225–239.

52 Spagnoletti, P., Kazermargi, N., Constantinides, P., and Prencipe, A. (2023). "Data control coordination in cloud-based ecosystems", in Handbook of Research on Digital Strategy, Cennamo, C., Dagnino, G.B., and Zhu, F. (eds.), Edward Elgar Publishing, pp. 289–307. Cheltenham and Camberley, UK.

53 See interesting article by Andrei Hagiu and Julian Wright https://platformchronicles.substack.com/p/when-pure-subscription-pricing-makes

54 Ibid.

55 Rivard, S., Lapointe, L. and Kappos, A., 2011. An organizational culture-based theory of clinical information systems implementation in hospitals. *Journal of the Association for Information Systems*, 12(2), p. 3; Lapointe, L. and Rivard, S., 2005. A multilevel model of resistance to information technology implementation. *MIS Quarterly*, 29(3), pp. 461–491; Constantinides, P. and Barrett, M., 2012. A narrative networks approach to understanding coordination practices in emergency response. *Information and organization*, 22(4), pp. 273–294.

56 Ibid.

57 Agarwal, R., Gao, G., DesRoches, C. and Jha, A.K., 2010. Research commentary—the digital transformation of healthcare: current status and the road ahead. *Information Systems Research*, 21(4), pp. 796–809; Rivard, S., Lapointe, L. and Kappos, A., 2011. An organizational culture-based theory of clinical information systems implementation in hospitals. *Journal of the Association for Information Systems*, 12(2), p. 3; Lapointe, L. and Rivard, S., 2005. A multilevel model of resistance to information technology implementation. *MIS Quarterly*, 29(3), pp. 461–491; Greenhalgh, T., Wherton, J., Papoutsi, C., Lynch, J., Hughes,

G., Hinder, S., Fahy, N., Procter, R. and Shaw, S., 2017. Beyond adoption: a new framework for theorizing and evaluating non-adoption, abandonment, and challenges to the scale-up, spread, and sustainability of health and care technologies. *Journal of Medical Internet Research*, 19(11), p. e367; Bhattacherjee, A. and Hikmet, N., 2007. Physicians' resistance toward healthcare information technology: a theoretical model and empirical test. *European Journal of Information Systems*, 16(6), pp. 725–737; Holden, R.J. and Karsh, B.T., 2010. The technology acceptance model: its past and its future in health care. *Journal of Biomedical Informatics*, 43(1), pp. 159–172; Kohli, R. and Kettinger, W.J., 2004. Informating the clan: controlling physicians' costs and outcomes. *MIS Quarterly*, 28(3), pp. 363–394; Constantinides, P. and Barrett, M., 2006. Negotiating ICT development and use: The case of a telemedicine system in the healthcare region of Crete. *Information and Organization*, 16(1), pp. 27–55.; Bernardi, R., Constantinides, P. and Nandhakumar, J., 2017. Challenging dominant frames in policies for IS innovation in healthcare through rhetorical strategies. *Journal of the Association for Information Systems*, 18(2), p. 3.

58 "Sideloading" apps mean installing apps that are not available on a platform's marketplace of apps from the web or alternative sources. While some marketplaces such as the Google Play Store allow sideloading, others such as the Apple App Store do not. See https://www.theverge.com/2021/11/3/22761724/apple-craig-federighi-ios-sideloading-web-summit-2021-european-commission-digital-markets-act

59 The most famous of these cases is that of Epic Games which sought to bypass Apple's strict pricing rules that do not allow apps to redirect their users off the platform to make in-app purchases. Epic Games claimed that purchases made by users inside its app should not incur the 30 percent tax (70/30 percent revenue share) by Apple. Apple claimed that this was already part of the contract and after a warning kicked Epic Games off the App Store. Epic Games took Apple to court and won; however, Apple has since appealed. See https://venturebeat.com/2021/09/10/epic-games-wins-injunction-favoring-alternative-payments-in-antitrust-lawsuit-against-apple/ and https://www.reuters.com/technology/us-appeals-court-pauses-antitrust-orders-against-apple-app-store-2021-12-08/

60 Tiwana, A., 2013. *Platform Ecosystems: Aligning Architecture, Governance, and Strategy*. Newnes; Zhang, Y., Li, J. and Tong, T.W., 2020. Platform governance matters: how platform gatekeeping affects knowledge sharing among complementors. *Strategic Management Journal*, 43(3), pp. 599–626.

61 See https://platformchronicles.substack.com/p/platform-leakage

62 Martens, B., Parker, G., Petropoulos, G. and Van Alstyne, M.W., 2021. Towards efficient information sharing in network markets. https://www.bruegel.org/2021/11/towards-efficient-information-sharing-in-network-markets/

63 Ibid.

64 Ibid. p. 4.

65 https://lifebit.ai/

66 Foerderer, J., Kude, T., Mithas, S. and Heinzl, A., 2018. Does platform owner's entry crowd out innovation? Evidence from Google photos. *Information Systems Research*, 29(2), pp. 444–460.

67 See interesting article by Andrei Hagiu and Julian Wright https://platformchronicles.substack.com/p/the-rise-of-roll-ups-on-amazon-and

68 Akerlof, G.A., 1978. The market for "lemons": Quality uncertainty and the market mechanism. *The Quarterly Journal of Economics*, 84(3), pp. 488–500; also see Cennamo, C., 2018. Building the value of next-generation platforms: the paradox of diminishing returns. *Journal of Management*, 44(8), pp. 3038–3069.

69 Hu, N., Bose, I., Koh, N.S. and Liu, L., 2012. Manipulation of online reviews: an analysis of ratings, readability, and sentiments. *Decision Support Systems*, 52(3), pp. 674–684; Mayzlin, D., Dover, Y. and Chevalier, J., 2014. Promotional reviews: an empirical investigation of online review manipulation. *American Economic Review*, 104(8), pp. 2421–2455.

70 Perrault, E.K. and Hildenbrand, G.M., 2020. The buffering effect of health care provider video biographies when viewed in combination with negative reviews: "you can't fake nice". *Journal of Medical Internet Research*, 22(4), p. e16635.

71 Vidanagama, D.U., Silva, T.P. and Karunananda, A.S., 2020. Deceptive consumer review detection: a survey. *Artificial Intelligence Review*, 53(2), pp. 1323–1352.

72 PatientsLikeMe was acquired by UnitedHealth Group in 2019 https://www.mobihealthnews.com/content/unitedhealth-group-acquires-patientslikeme

73 CorEvitas, previously called Corona, acquired HealthUnlocked https://www.corevitas.com/news/corrona-acquires-healthunlocked-creating-first-class-patient-experience-ecosystem

74 See for example https://hbr.org/2020/10/how-to-thrive-when-everything-feels-terrible

75 See study on HealthUnlocked by Costello, R.E., Anand, A., Evans, M.J. and Dixon, W.G., 2019. Associations between engagement with an online health community and changes in patient activation and health care utilization: longitudinal web-based survey. *Journal of Medical Internet Research*, 21(8), p. e13477; also relevant study on PatientsLikeMe by Wicks, P., Massagli, M., Frost, J., Brownstein, C., Okun, S., Vaughan, T., Bradley, R. and Heywood, J., 2010. Sharing health data for better outcomes on PatientsLikeMe. *Journal of Medical Internet Research*, 12(2), p. e1549.

76 Frost, J. and Massagli, M., 2008. Social uses of personal health information within PatientsLikeMe, an online patient community: what can happen when patients have access to one another's data. *Journal of Medical Internet Research*, 10(3), p. e15.

77 Ibid.

78 See press report on the ecosystem collaboration between The Mighty and pharma companies https://www.pharmaceutical-technology.com/features/the-mighty-patients-pharma-social-media/

79 See video case study here https://www.youtube.com/watch?v=JAphgrgP_tA&t=31s

5   Blockchain Infrastructures in Healthcare

In recent years, blockchain infrastructures have emerged as more efficient, distributed and secure solutions to the challenge of data silos, including the associated challenge of securing the privacy of patient data. Although blockchain infrastructures are no silver bullet to solving the data challenge, they can provide distributed mechanisms to enable secluded healthcare organizations operating in data silos to achieve not only inter-operable but also trustworthy exchanges of medical data.

Prior to blockchain infrastructures, actors in an ecosystem relied on third parties to establish trust and to mitigate risks in transactions.[1] Traditionally, trusted third parties have been the central node in a centralized infrastructure. This allows for uniformity of connection and validation, but at the cost of a single point of delay or failure in the centralized node. The key benefits of such a centralized approach are that trusted third parties can validate identities and ownership of data resources, while each actor in an ecosystem maintains its own database management system.[2] In addition, each actor can unilaterally execute decisions about accounting rules, transaction reversals, software upgrades and so on, within their own organizational boundaries.[3]

Despite these benefits, however, centralized infrastructures via trusted third parties provide little transparency of transactions outside each actor's organizational bounda-ries. For actors interacting within a broader ecosystem, this immediately becomes problematic. The interdependencies between ecosystem actors become very difficult to coordinate, and a number of collective action problems emerge. For example, records of transactions are mutable; there is nothing to prevent ecosystem actors from modifying these records after transactions have been executed. There is also a risk of "vendor opportunism",[4] where third-party complementors may pursue their self-interests, while not complying with the terms and conditions of the agreement. Therefore, ecosystem actors spend a lot of resources monitoring agreements to make sure that all are behaving as promised. In the event of disputes and conflicts of interest, reconciliations become expensive and time-consuming.[5] In addition, the cost of transactions is very high because of the control and fees claimed by the trusted third parties. Finally, each actor has to spend significant resources to secure transactions within their independent organiza-tional boundaries.

Blockchain infrastructures were initially developed to challenge traditional financial models that are heavily dependent on trusted third parties such as banks. In such financial models, the banks are meant to address the "double-spending problem", that is, the possibility that a coin is spent twice by the same actor.[6] Banks act as trusted third parties to keep records for every account and to trace and verify every claimed transaction. Although these traditional models can be efficient and convenient, the

DOI: 10.4324/9781032619569-7

aforementioned collective action problems eventually led to the development of a new type of cryptocurrency, namely, Bitcoin, to remove the need of a centralized trusted third party.[7]

Since the introduction of Bitcoin, blockchain infrastructures have become a new approach to solving the collective action problems related to recording, tracking, validating and aggregating various types of assets, and especially data, across fields and applications, including healthcare.[8]

This chapter discusses ways by which healthcare organizations can form ecosystems on blockchain infrastructures. The chapter describes how blockchain infrastructures work, how transactions take place and how they enable distributed data governance. It then provides a discussion of use cases of blockchain infrastructures in healthcare provided by PharmaLedger,[9] focusing on recruiting patients and achieving informed consent in clinical trials, and achieving trusted transactions through electronic product information (ePI) in pharmaceutical supply chains. The chapter concludes by discussing the co-innovation and co-adoption challenges of the use of blockchain infrastructures in healthcare.

5.1 A New Approach to Distributed Data Governance in Healthcare

5.1.1 Transactions on Blockchain Infrastructures

Blockchain infrastructures are distributed ledger technologies that provide a shared, immutable record of transactions between ecosystem actors. Instead of centralized trusted third parties, ecosystem actors achieve mutual trust through consensus algorithms that set the terms and conditions for transactions to occur.[10]

Consensus is a computer science problem of making a network of computers distributed over the Internet agree on a value in the presence of faults. This problem was first articulated as the "Byzantine Generals Problem",[11] whereby a group of generals have surrounded a city, but can only take it if they all attack at once. If they do not all attack at once, they run the risk of failure, while suffering heavy losses. There are also traitors who are actively trying to subvert the generals' efforts, so coordination between the generals is needed. The key idea behind the Byzantine consensus is that we can devise mechanisms that can tolerate not just computers in a network failing but we can also actually tolerate malicious adversaries on the network who might be trying to subvert agreement.

Since the Byzantine consensus was articulated, there have been many different types of consensus algorithms developed, many of which are still being used to control the scheduling of data centers in many different organizations across sectors.[12] For example, the proof of work (PoW) consensus algorithm is used in Bitcoin blockchain to prove the authenticity of any block that is added to the blockchain. A considerable amount of computing power is required to do the work which provides a financial incentive in the form of Bitcoins. The transactions are verified by every computer node in the network and rejected as invalid if faulty transactions are included in the block. This process of verifying Bitcoin transactions and storing them in blockchain is called mining. The miner is the actor who solves the PoW puzzle to validate the transaction. In the past, individual actors would use their home computers to mine Bitcoins. However, as Bitcoin became more valuable, miners joined forces and started purchasing specialized mining hardware called application-specific integrated circuits to solve the PoW puzzle millions of times faster than individual actors could. So, in the last decade or so, a whole industry of

Bitcoin miners has spawned, raising questions around electricity consumption and the concentration of mining by powerful groups, among other issues.[13]

Exactly because of the negative implications of mining, alternative consensus algorithms have been developed. For example, proof of stake (PoS) consensus algorithms also use incentives, but instead of monetary rewards they assign voting rights based on the amount of money actors have in the blockchain. Agreement is reached based on the proportion of stake that actors have and that is why it is called proof of stake. For example, "if Alice, Bob and Carol's stakes are 500, 300 and 200 coins, respectively, then Alice will be selected as the validator 50% of the time and Bob and Carol 30% and 20% of the time, respectively".[14] Thus, the more stake actors have, the more likely they will be selected as the validator and receive the financial reward. Although PoS algorithms have different incentives from those of PoW such as reducing the need for expensive hardware and increased computational power while also reducing electricity consumption, they also suffer from a number of negative externalities such as actors with high stakes becoming even more wealthy while repeatedly excluding actors with smaller stakes.[15]

Another related consensus algorithm is delegated proof of stake (DPoS) where actors use their stake to vote for validators or delegate their voting power to another actor. Selected validators are responsible for creating blocks by verifying transactions. If they verify and sign all transactions in a block, they receive a reward, which is usually shared with those who have voted for them. Votes are proportionate to the size of each voter's stake. However, actors acting as validators need not have a large stake to enter the competition. Rather, votes from actors with large stakes can result in actors with relatively small stakes being elevated to a higher tier. Still the DPoS consensus is susceptible to coercion and weighted voting that again may benefit a select few actors. Evidently, no matter what consensus algorithm is being used, there are trade-offs.

These consensus algorithms sit at the very core of a blockchain infrastructure and drive the transactions between a set of actors in a digital platform ecosystem such as the ones described in Chapter 4. Actors that form this digital platform ecosystem use consensus algorithms to agree on blocks that form a blockchain infrastructure. Those blocks could refer to data on financial transactions or information transactions such as accessing and storing EHRs. So, for example, if a doctor at a hospital requests access to an EHR on the blockchain, this request is broadcasted to other actors in the platform ecosystem. These actors validate the received transaction request based on already established consensus algorithms. If validated, the transaction is added to a newly created block or it is added to an existing block with other validated transactions. The new or modified block becomes part of the blockchain infrastructure and the database is updated with copies shared with all actors in the platform ecosystem. Every single actor on the platform ecosystem can construct an auditable verifiable database view of this blockchain infrastructure. The reason that this database is auditable and verifiable is because cryptography hash functions and digital signatures[16] are used in order to enable actors to verify all the data that have been added to the blockchain. All actors use the same blockchain and so everyone gets a copy of it every time a new block is added or an existing block is modified. In turn, this makes the blockchain immutable and trustworthy. Depending on the type of blockchain, the transaction validation and block creation tasks are driven by consensus competitions that are incentivized by monetary or non-monetary rewards. Figure 5.1 summarizes this process.

As evident from Figure 5.1, unlike centralized database management systems, in which data is controlled by a single trusted third party, in a blockchain infrastructure,

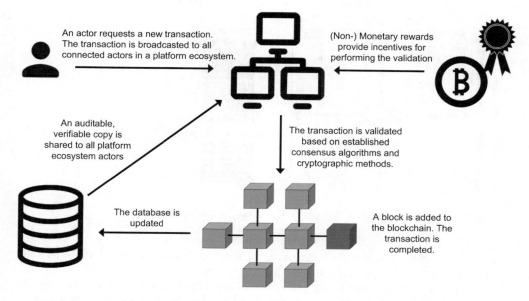

Figure 5.1 A Transaction Process on a Blockchain Infrastructure with everyone having an audited copy of the process.

multiple parties validate or reject transactions. Control over transactions is distributed among several independent actors who can make updates to the blockchain and interact directly without the need to rely on central coordination.[17]

5.1.2   Degrees of (De)Centralization in Blockchain Infrastructures

At this point, it becomes important to differentiate between different degrees of (de)centralization because it will help clarify *when* a blockchain infrastructure will be necessary and valuable to a healthcare ecosystem. There are two axes, namely, *architectural (de)centralization* and *governance (de)centralization*.[18] These axes align with the digital transformation framework presented in Chapter 4, in relation to different types of architectures and governance mechanisms. Figure 5.2 provides an illustration of these axes while placing different types of infrastructure across these.

First, **architectural (de)centralization** refers to *the degree of (de)centralization of the technological infrastructure of blockchain*. This infrastructure is built on a modular layered architecture that can be broadly abstracted as including an *application layer*, that provides a user interface and defines the business logic and various services (including smart contracts) that can interact with the database; the *data layer*, that contains the blockchain data structures (i.e., where the transactions and blocks are created); the *consensus layer* where cryptographic protocols like PoW and PoS are executed; and finally, the *network layer* represented by the computer nodes that make up the computational power to participate in the consensus layer, validating or rejecting new transactions and storing the whole history of the transactions on the database.[19] Each of these layers can be proprietary or open and tightly or loosely coupled, thus pointing at a spectrum of architecture (de)centralization. The data and application layers are usually "off-chain" to ensure higher

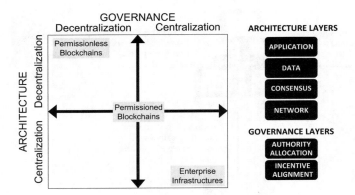

Figure 5.2 Decentralized vs Centralized Blockchain Infrastructures.

speed and scalability, whereas the consensus and network layers are "on-chain" and thus bound to the blockchain (see Figure 5.1).[20]

Second, **governance (de)centralization** refers to *the degree of (de)centralization of the governance structures of blockchain.* As discussed in Chapter 4, governance is achieved through incentive alignment and authority allocation (i.e., control).[21] Authority allocation refers to various decisions rights over the blockchain, whereas incentive alignment refers to monetary and non-monetary rewards that aim at aligning actor behavior with the architectural design. These can be implemented through peer-to-peer and inter-organizational agreements or through automated, machine learning technologies.

Although there is a spectrum of (de)centralization models,[22] three key models can be defined along the axes of architecture and governance, as seen in Figure 5.2.

At the bottom right corner of the figure, a central actor or a collective of actors acts as a trusted third party with full control over proprietary architectural layers. Just like in the case of tightly coupled, proprietary-based platform architectures discussed in Chapter 4, incentives will be based on arms-length relationships between the trusted third party, who acts as an orchestrator and the rest of the ecosystem actors. In this model, a blockchain is not needed, and an enterprise infrastructure controlled by a trusted third party can address the needs of all actors.

Blockchain infrastructures are several degrees more decentralized than enterprise infrastructures and are often distinguished as public vs private and permissioned vs permissionless.[23] Public blockchains allow all actors in a platform ecosystem to read data from the blockchain and request and validate new transactions, whereas private blockchains allow only actors who have been preregistered by a central authority to do all the aforementioned actions. Public blockchains can be built with either permissioned or permissionless configurations for transaction validation, whereas private blockchains can only be built on permissioned ones.

As seen in Figure 5.2, permissionless blockchains sit at the upper left corner because they point at both a decentralized architecture with open layers and a decentralized governance whereby no actor has control or authority over the others. Rather, governance is achieved through monetary rewards in the form of cryptocurrencies, while actors engage in PoW competitions that require extensive computational power to solve complex mathematical puzzles. The complexity helps address security problems in a large crowd of anonymous actors. Since the first permissionless blockchain was developed to transfer digital tokens in the form of Bitcoins, other permissionless blockchains such as Ethereum emerged to allow more sophisticated transactions through smart contracts that execute pre-coded pieces of software on the blockchain when specific conditions are met.[24] Smart contracts can execute transactions autonomously, without approval from third parties, and could potentially manifest in machine-to-machine coordination over the Internet of Things.[25] Permissionless blockchains are preferred when transactions can be crowdsourced to a large unidentified group of actors, as in the case of mining for Bitcoins and other cryptocurrencies. In those cases, having a central authority can actually create problems of power accumulation and lack of transparency in the transactions.

In contrast, permissioned blockchains are preferred when roles need to be defined in advance, identities verified and access is secured. Permissioned blockchains are not anonymous and are usually developed by private entities like healthcare organizations, where some level of trust is already established between participating parties. So, permissioned blockchains restrict access to a predefined group of actors whose identity is known to everyone in the blockchain and who have voting rights in the transactions. Because of this, permissioned blockchains usually employ consensus algorithms such as PoS and DPoS and relevant incentives around non-monetary awards.

Although there are different levels of access, in both permissionless and permissioned blockchains, decision rights over the functionality of the core infrastructure and its components, how those can be executed and who has control will often be implemented in the design of the blockchain itself, as opposed to being written in arms-length contract agreements.[26] For example, who has *read*, *submit* and *validate* rights over transactions will often be integrated into smart contracts and executed automatically by software agents. These rights will vary depending on the underlying consensus algorithms. In addition, when there is disagreement over the decision-making about a transaction request, a fork is created, meaning that a block is split in two. In permissionless blockchains where the software that runs on the different layers is most often open source, forks are created to fix security issues or reverse transactions that are found to be in breach of established rules or to have malicious intent. Forks may also be created when there is disagreement over the cryptographic techniques and underlying consensus algorithm upon which transactions are carried out. Such so-called "hard" forks[27] can lead to the development of completely new blockchains.[28] It is for this reason that permissioned blockchains seem to still benefit from "benevolent dictatorship"[29] governance structures. This point aligns well with the discussion in Chapter 4 around the benefits of having an ecosystem orchestrator, who is in a better position to coordinate value-capture and value-creation opportunities as opposed to completely decentralizing decision rights among participating ecosystem actors.

This categorization of different types of infrastructures, based on degrees of architecture and governance (de)centralization, brings to the surface the importance of clarifying the conditions of a possible blockchain implementation. Not all ecosystems will require a blockchain infrastructure. In fact, many will do just fine without one. There are some key underlying conditions that need to be met for an ecosystem to select a blockchain infrastructure, and this infrastructure may only fulfill a part of an ecosystem's digital transformation such as validating a patient's digital identity and providing access to patient data.

Academics[30] and consultants[31] have proposed a set of conditions that need to be met to select a blockchain infrastructure. These can be summarized as follows. A blockchain infrastructure is necessary when(a) *multiple actors generate transactions that change information in a commonly shared database,*(b) *those actors have conflicts of interest over the information being changed such that centrally enforced governance rules are not possible,* (c)*intermediaries are not efficient or in a position to act as arbiters of truth* and (d)*security over the integrity and verifiability of the database is compromised.*

These conditions can actually translate to the key value propositions of a blockchain infrastructure. First, a blockchain infrastructure enables multiple actors to access a commonly shared database that produces immutable records for all. Second, it provides distributed governance structures that can address potential conflicts of interest. Third, it replaces intermediaries with consensus algorithms and cryptographic techniques that act as arbiters of truth. Finally, it secures the integrity and verifiability of the commonly shared database.

Now that the broad value propositions, possible technological architectures and governance structures of blockchain have been described, we can examine how these apply in real-world use cases in healthcare ecosystems.

5.2   Use Cases of Blockchain Infrastructures in Healthcare Ecosystems

This section explores use cases of blockchain infrastructures provided by PharmaLedger.[32] PharmaLedger was a European Commission Innovative Medicines Initiative (IMI), supported by the European Federation of Pharmaceutical Industries and Associations. The PharmaLedger Project was comprised of 29 organizations overall. These come from a range of backgrounds that include pharma, small-to-medium technology enterprises, academic institutes and patient and healthcare organizations. PharmaLedger has developed blockchain technologies across different domains and is now continuing its work through an independent not-for-profit, the PharmaLedger Association (PLA). The next subsections briefly discuss two of these domains, namely, recruiting patients and achieving informed consent in clinical trials, and achieving trusted transactions through ePI in pharmaceutical supply chains. This discussion draws on publicly available documents and reports from the PharmaLedger project.[33]

5.2.1   Use Case 1: Blockchain for Clinical Trials

One of the most promising areas of applying blockchain infrastructures is in the management of personal patient data. Although regulations such as the GDPR and HIPAA can cover a wider set of data types than has previously been the case with data protection legislation, much of this data is centrally governed by third parties that make such regulation potentially impractical. The study by the *Financial Times*[34] that was described in Chapter 2, whereby data from parenting site Babycentre was tracked by third-party companies around the Internet and especially by Google's advertising arm DoubleClick, illustrates the scale and risks of the problem. The privacy and confidentiality of personal patient data is being compromised on these digital platform ecosystems without much transparency as to who processes such data.

Processing is broadly understood to mean *any activities such as collecting, recording, organizing, structuring, storing, using and erasing data, regardless of whether any of these is done by automated means or manually.*[35] Processing of personal data is lawful when the data subject has given consent.[36]

Consent is defined as *"any freely given, specific, informed and unambiguous indication of the data subject's wishes by which he or she, by a statement or by a clear* *affirmative action, signifies agreement to the processing of personal data relating to him or her".*[37] Consent presupposes that individual persons are offered a genuine choice about the terms of the intended processing activity over their personal data, or declining them without detriment[38] (e.g., they can still get access to a service even if they choose not to consent to certain processing activities).

Personal data covers *"any information relating to an identified or identifiable natural person".*[39] Persons can be identified, directly or indirectly, in particular by reference to an identifier such as a name, an identification number, location data, an online identifier (e.g., IP address, browser cookies) or to one or more factors specific to the physical, physiological, genetic, mental, economic, cultural or social identity of that natural person.[40] Although one piece of data does not directly identify someone, relevance is usually established by combining that data with data held separately elsewhere. Because of this data linking, a distinctive profile of an individual may be created.[41]

One way to ensure the privacy and confidentiality of personal patient data is to use blockchain infrastructures designed to align with regulations such as GDPR and HIPAA. Participants on a blockchain network have unique personal addresses that are shared on the blockchain. These addresses comprise a series of random alphanumeric characters that make up the public key to the participant's account. The public key is linked to a private key known solely by the participant. Data encrypted with the public key can only be decrypted with the private key, and vice versa. Public–private key pairs are randomly generated by participants in their digital wallets. Digital wallets are software applications that run on personal devices or desktop computers. Unless public keys are linked to additional information that can reveal the identity behind the key, individuals remain anonymous to the rest of the blockchain participants.

Blockchain infrastructures can help achieve self-sovereign identities[42] while meeting such regulatory principles as anonymity, data minimization[43] and data security. Patient data has traditionally been managed by healthcare service providers not by the patients themselves. The idea behind self-sovereign identities is that users should own and control their identities along with all of the data-related attributes associated with those identities. Users should control their identity in a digital wallet that contains verifiable claims like medical records and degree certificates, and these claims can be trusted across healthcare ecosystems, by service providers, payers and other ecosystem actors. Blockchain infrastructures enable a model of self-sovereign identity to work.

From a privacy perspective, there are several benefits of this model of digital, self-sovereign identities. First, verifying identity attributes can be done while using a zero-knowledge proof mechanism,[44] which makes it possible to prove an attribute without disclosing or revealing any additional information, thus preserving anonymity. For example, patients can prove that they are older than 18 years of age without disclosing their date of birth. Another point is that identity attributes can also be limited to the absolute minimum necessary, thus achieving data minimization. For example, patients can disclose their age, blood type and health vitals in different claims. Third, verifiable claims can be exchanged off-chain by using encrypted and secure channels, thus ensuring data security.

Building on the above principles, PharmaLedger developed a use case to pre-screen patients for clinical trials, while leveraging blockchain as a shared ledger of patient permissions accessible by multiple parties without any single party in charge. The platform can be used by all sponsors, regulators, ethics committees and site labs, offering the ability to improve compliance and traceability, automate procedures, increase efficiency, and provide real-time visibility of consent and enrollment status to the relevant stakeholders while maintaining privacy.

One of the key challenges in conducting clinical trials for research and development of new drugs and treatments is recruiting individuals who want to voluntarily participate and meet the criteria for inclusion. Each clinical trial has a careful set of criteria for who can participate. Discussions happen between the patient and the doctor at a clinical site and the doctor explains the study, the benefits and the risks. Research shows that 80 percent of trials fail to meet the enrolment timelines,[45] and this is due primarily because of the use of study-centric recruitment methods, where individuals are recruited on the basis of whether they meet the study criteria. The current process followed in recruiting patients for clinical trials is not friendly for patients; it is also very costly and inefficient. It is also prone to generate duplication, while data is locked in silos.

PharmaLedger developed a patient-centric recruitment platform, where patients provide their medical history and consent to have their data used to match them to clinical trials. The platform aggregates clinical trials and screens criteria across multiple studies and sponsors, while using an algorithm to match patients to relevant clinical trials. Patients get notified of any matches and they share their contact information with clinical sites so they can follow up for a full screening and enrollment in the clinical trial. The general principle is to allow patients to manually input their health data or connect to a data source such as an electronic medical record to have their anonymized data matched to clinical trials. To access the PharmaLedger Clinical Trial Recruitment platform, involved stakeholders (patients, physicians, sponsors and clinical sites) must create accounts by providing sign-up credentials (full name, email address and password). Patients' health data is captured in their digital wallet (self-sovereign application) and sharing of this data can happen only if the patient takes an active role to enable sharing through the dynamic permissioning capability of the PharmaLedger solution.

Through an eConsent application, patients are informed about the objectives of a clinical trial study after which they can choose to provide their consent to voluntarily participate in the study. After the informed consent form has been signed, the patient then gets screened to confirm their eligibility. Their data gets collected and evaluated in relation to the clinical trial's objectives. Then, this data gets shared with only the appropriate permission users that are participating in the study. Currently, the informed consent and the risk processes are done through a manual process. Research has shown that over 50 percent of clinical trials fail in clinical development with 57 percent of those failing due to inadequate efficacy.[46] Blockchain technology can help improve protocol compliance, the completeness of data and the quality of the clinical trial process. By incorporating informed consent in the process, blockchain technology can add immutability, automation, trust and real-time updates. Trial participants are informed in detail not only about the purpose of the study and its procedures but also about the risks of participating in the study, as well as the benefits. There is also a disclosure of alternative procedures, if any, that could be beneficial for the participant.

5.2.2   Use Case 2: Blockchain for Pharmaceutical Supply Chains

The second use case focuses on the creation of ePI of pharmaceutical supplies in digital form. Relevant ecosystem actors include product manufacturers, pharmaceutical companies, health regulatory authorities, patients and healthcare providers.

Currently, most drugs and other pharmaceutical supplies come with paper leaflets that explain how those supplies should be used, their known side effects and risks. Ironically, this information is electronically produced but then printed and added into the supply package. The limitations are well recognized, including low readability because of the small print, limited language options and a lag between the provision of new information as the print and physical supply takes time to update through the supply chain. There are also environmental concerns due to the billions of leaflets printed in the industry each year.

ePI can be produced in a format suitable for authoring, review, approval and dissemination using blockchain technology. Manufacturers can obtain their own unique enterprise wallet, where they can store thousands of electronic leaflets for thousands of different products. Furthermore, updates can be made through the enterprise wallet without delay. As soon as the updated leaflet is approved by the health authorities, that would be updated also in the manufacturers' enterprise wallets.

The end-users, whether they are patients or healthcare providers, can access these ePI by using a mobile application on personal devices such as their smartphones. They can scan the datamatrix barcode on the product package, and the backend technology of the blockchain resolver will find the correct manufacturer's enterprise wallet for the product. The end-users can immediately access the most up-to-date leaflet. Instant access with the most up-to-date leaflet are key benefits of this technology.

The datamatrix barcode has three key bits of information. The global trade identification number, the serial number, and the batch number, all of which are important for tracing and updating product information. For example, if a manufacturer has a batch recall, they can add that date into their enterprise wallet and when a patient or a healthcare professional scan the code, they will get a message that the product is recalled. This can help improve safety. The metadata and services accessed through this system can be expanded to deliver other important data and information across the ecosystem including two-factor authentication of the product, serial number and anti-counterfeit feature, as well as finished good traceability features and adverse event reporting among others. For example, the anti-counterfeit check can verify that the package is legitimate and can be traced back to a manufacturer in the ecosystem. This can help improve trust among ecosystem parners. It is also possible to use the barcode and the app for adverse event reporting. When a pharmaceutical product is released to the market, the regulatory authorities continue to monitor their advocacy and safety throughout the product's life. If a patient experiences an adverse event of a product, they are encouraged to report that back to the regulatory authorities who can help with policy decisions and with improving the information on the leaflets.

This use case requires the PharmaLedger platform to implement a number of compliance measures required by, for example, the EU Annex 11 on GxP Computerized Systems[47] and the US FDA21CFR820 on Quality Management of GxP systems.[48] Just like the first use case, it also needs to meet the requirements of several privacy legislations including the EU GDPR around its data privacy management system. Given that manufacturers could be located anywhere in the world, compliance with local regulation and data privacy legislation will vary, and this poses one of the key challenges faced by the PharmaLedger platform.

PharmaLedger uses a vendor agnostic infrastructure based on the OpenDSU technology standard.[49] This means that the PharmaLedger platform can form a layered hierarchy of blockchains, whereby data stored in higher layer blockchains is cryptographically anchored on parent blockchains, whose data is in turn anchored on their parents and so on. The lower layer in the hierarchy is a PharmaLedger root blockchain. This ensures higher levels of security, traceability and verification of integrity and authenticity. A blockchain naming service is provided to facilitate addressing entities throughout the PharmaLedger blockchain hierarchy. Higher layer blockchains are independent of each other and may use different blockchain protocols. They may use minimal smart contracts to anchor their data on their parent blockchain and support anchoring of data from their branched blockchains.

Typically, a dedicated blockchain serves each PharmaLedger use case. Other functions that serve the entire PharmaLedger blockchain ecosystem may also be implemented on dedicated blockchains (such as decentralized identity management). At the same time, it is possible to switch a PharmaLedger application to a different blockchain infrastructure and protocol, without changing the application code. This can be done by changing only wrappers and APIs. Within a blockchain dedicated to a specific use case, an arbitrary implementation can be used. For example, a use case may be implemented using a blockchain from the Ethereum blockchain family, while using no or minimal smart contracts, while another use case may be implemented on HyperLedger Fabric and rely heavily on chaincode.

Each dedicated blockchain follows the principle of minimization of code and data implemented and stored on-chain. Data sharing units (DSUs) implement the business logic of use cases and store off-chain data. DSUs contain self-sovereign code and data and are executed in user-controlled execution environments using client-side encryption and user wallets.[50] These wallets, at a minimum, store private keys and facilitate making blockchain transactions but may implement also other arbitrary functions.

Standard APIs such as REST are used for interfacing with external applications. For example, APIs may be used for interfacing with legacy health applications, non-PharmaLedger use cases or external blockchains. PharmaLedger libraries, tools and SDK are provided to simplify application development. The technology agnostic nature of the PharmaLedger platform benefits use-case specific deployments. The main function of the platform is security and hierarchical anchoring of data, with self-sovereign code and data stored mainly off-chain and with dedicated blockchains for use cases and major functions.

5.3   Co-Innovation and Co-Adoption Challenges

The PharmaLedger ecosystem has been developed using European research funds and supported by the European Commission IMI, as described earlier. As such, although very innovative and exhibiting the great potential of utilizing blockchain to achieve not only interoperable but also trustworthy exchanges of data, there is a real challenge of sustaining the ecosystem after the funds run out. In fact, a recent review of blockchain projects in healthcare has found that although many of these projects appear successful none have moved beyond the proof-of-concept stage,[51] something which points to low digital maturity.

Similarly, although there is wide agreement that the two use cases discussed above are feasible and could generate great value for ecosystem partners,[52] actual implementations of these two use cases are not easy. As the previous sections have pointed out, the architecture of these blockchain technologies is complex, requiring radical transformation of existing business processes and operations and a change in people mindsets and the ways they work. More importantly, there needs to be a high level of ecosystem-wide commitment and trust to develop the governance rules required to manage blockchain transactions.

No doubt, once the infrastructure is in place and the governance agreed, the benefits to be realized will exceed those of more conventional technologies. However, getting there will require addressing a number of co-innovation and co-adoption challenges.

As evident from the two use cases described above, co-innovating blockchain technologies resembles open-source technology projects that utilize vendor-agnostic, loosely coupled components. The ecosystem orchestrator is usually a community or consortium of organizations that has a limited ability to enforce common governance rules; therefore, the transformation project may run into coordination and integration issues before it lifts off. Permissioned blockchains will be used to define ecosystem roles in advance, while restricting access to a predefined group of actors whose identity is known to everyone in the blockchain and who have voting rights in the transactions. However, deciding who has what rights over transactions will be challenged by participating actors.

In relation to the first use case of managing clinical trial data, most pharmaceutical companies will want to act as ecosystem orchestrators of a given blockchain infrastructure and to control that data. The reality is that it costs billions to develop new drugs, and pharmaceutical companies want a return on their investment.[53] Research has shown that pharmaceutical companies not only fund and help design clinical trials for specific types of drugs, but they also influence the promotion and adoption of these drugs by sponsoring the researchers and doctors who prescribe them.[54] Clinical trial data could be used to identify new studies, repurpose existing drugs and develop new ones, while protecting any intellectual property rights that emerge in the process. Thus, the incentive structures are such that pharmaceutical companies would want to orchestrate their own ecosystems and control innovation. This would kill all the value propositions of a blockchain infrastructure from the outset.

There is an incentive for small pharmaceutical companies to join forces and to share anonymous clinical trial data that they would otherwise not have access to because of limited funds. Joining an ecosystem would also protect these smaller companies from hostile takeovers or acquisitions, depending on the founders' exit strategies. This would ensure fairer competition in a market dominated by big pharmaceutical companies.[55] Joining an ecosystem would enable more robust data access and better patient recruitment into clinical trials for these smaller pharmaceutical companies. If they were to go about it on their own, they would have to face recruitment costs ranging between US$2 billion and US$3 billion, something which could force them to seek help from bigger sponsors.[56] Patient data would be aggregated, anonymized and subject to patient-driven permissions, something that would allow these smaller pharmaceutical companies to share resources.

Still, the shared governance of the clinical trial data and the overall process would have to be negotiated and agreed upon prior to building the blockchain technology. For example, data integrity and data provenance have to be established with regulatory authorities to help ensure that clinical results maintain their integrity throughout the process. The eConsent application proposed by PharmaLedger can certainly develop a built-in layer of transparency and traceability by time-stamping each step of a patient's consent and potentially automating it via set rules in smart contracts. However, the study protocols still need to be defined and established among the ecosystem actors in time for a regulatory inquiry.[57]

In relation to the second use case, pharmaceutical supply chains are complex and often involve trading partners in several different countries, with operations subject to different trade, legal and regulatory regimes.[58] Establishing interoperability between the technology infrastructures of the various ecosystem actors involved including manufacturers, wholesalers, repackagers, logistic providers, regulators, hospitals and pharmacies would require collective agreement or a benevolent dictator to enforce common standards and interfaces. Governance becomes critical once again. Specifically, who will participate in the blockchain infrastructure, how will data be validated and how will confidential supply chain data be shared among participants will need to be predefined. Many of the collective action problems discussed in Chapter 4 will apply here, and these problems will vary depending on the digital maturity of ecosystem participants. Although blockchain technology can automate many governance mechanisms through smart contracts, still the actual mechanisms would have to be agreed upon by ecosystem participants. If these are not collectively agreed, then the actual blockchain technology cannot be built.

A recent survey of 300 manufacturers, distributors and retailers noted that the co-adoption of blockchain technologies into pharmaceutical supply chains is very slow because of low buy-in and acceptance, poor integration into existing supply chain networks, but also the significant amount of training needed to develop human capabilities.[59] The cost of adoption and implementation is a key challenge for ecosystem actors as these blockchain solutions may not inherently drive revenue and benefits may take time to realize. For example, although electronic health records (EHRs) are now required to have patient-facing APIs in many countries, the same is not true for other types of data, especially supply chain data. Incentivizing ecosystem actors to build data connections without clear, financial benefits is challenging, and this is exactly the difference between compliance and true interoperability. Actors may comply to new regulation, but making their systems and data interoperable will require other types of incentives.

In addition to the aforementioned organizational challenges, there are a number of technical challenges that need to be addressed. Although private permissioned blockchains are the best option for a number of use cases in healthcare, most of these blockchains are prone to a 51% attack, where a single entity can gain control of the majority of the network.[60] This happens because, unlike public permissionless blockchains that have thousands of participants, in a private permissioned blockchain, the central trustworthy nodes become more compromised by possible attackers. Since the validation of the transactions is centralized (e.g., in the case of clinical trials this is done by the sponsor(s)), the attacker may gain the authority to control the computational power of the network, causing a transaction to happen twice. Hence, the integrity of the transaction data is affected and the resources of the network are exhausted. This has negative implications on the integrity of the data and service availability, which are critical for healthcare applications.[61]

Furthermore, the feasibility of using blockchain in healthcare is dependent on the technology capabilities of storing and processing vast amounts of patient data, while ensuring the privacy and security of the data and reducing operating costs.[62] To achieve such technology capabilities, private permissioned blockchain technologies need to be customized to fit the needs of the specific use cases, something that may result in compromising some of the principles of blockchain technology.[63] This is a known trade-off when innovating new blockchain solutions in healthcare.[64] For instance, complying with GDPR requirements involves compromising the immutability of blockchain. PharmaLedger has implemented detailed guidance from CNIL to comply with GDPR while maintaining immutability by destruction of private keys.[65]

Additionally, the block size limitation in blockchain is intended to reduce performance overhead and prevent DDoS attacks. However, this compromises the scalability needed to accommodate the vast amount of patient data.[66] What makes blockchain unique is the ability of all actors to verify and validate who is accessing which data and for what purpose. However, if every computer in the blockchain network has to verify every step of every smart contract, efficiency and scalability will be hurt. If the blockchain is designed to process large data, it will cause extra operating costs due to the performance overhead, and it will expose the network to DDoS attacks. Blockchain technologies would also be difficult to upgrade in order to fix a bug or to respond to an attack, because in each of these cases there would need to be agreement by all participants. Developers will not have the ability to just push out an update before that is validated by the ecosystem.

One solution to the above problems is to assign committees that would take on the responsibility of acting on behalf of the ecosystem, instead of having everyone voting and participating in these governance decisions. Governance can be nested such that, some committees act as general-purpose structures to organize decisions across different task divisions, whereas others act as more specialized structures to organize decisions within a task division. The higher layer can supervise decisions at lower layers. In doing so, they can address horizontal assurance problems that may arise in relation to who is accessing which data and for what purpose. This nesting of governance mechanisms can ensure that all actors with a substantive interest in a particular data domain and task division are represented adequately.[67] This nesting of governance can be technically enforced with what is called "sharding", which is the division of data so that different groups of participants in the blockchain take a portion of the data transactions to validate and secure.

More recently, the PLA, a global not-for-profit organization, was legally formed in March 2022 in Basel, Switzerland, as the sustainability strategy of the PharmaLedger Project. "PLA is a pre-competition umbrella organization dedicated to the development and deployment of trusted solutions for the healthcare ecosystem. PLA is the neutral venue where all healthcare players can collaborate, pool resources, and share risks associated with the development of Healthcare 4.0 solutions".[68] The PLA is meant to act as a meta-organizing body that can orchestrate multiple ecosystems on the open-source, vendor-agnostic infrastructure described in section 5.2.2. The PLA has implemented a nested governance structure as discussed above, whereby product teams that are open to all members take accountability for each product area. These are then overseen by technical, quality and management committees to ensure not only strategic alignment and regulatory compliance but also effective governance of ecosystem interactions.

Related to but separate from privacy and security is the challenge of patient engagement.[69] A patient-driven, blockchain interoperability framework necessarily involves more patient participation than if the patient was engaged via a single healthcare organization such as a hospital. If a patient receives care at one hospital, and they seek outside records from another organization, a patient may simply sign a form, and their healthcare providers will facilitate the exchange. However, for patients to effectively manage their own data and other digital assets on a blockchain, they would need additional support and training. This would involve storing their data safely with passwords and encryption keys. Patients will have varied digital capabilities, and many will require someone to do this for them. It is not immediately clear who would play this role, but there is an opportunity for new types of digital platforms, akin to cryptocurrency exchanges. Such digital platforms could be designed along nested governance structures as discussed above.

Evidently, there are many different types of challenges in co-innovating and co-adopting blockchain technologies. There are technical challenges around how many actors (i.e., nodes) should be included in a blockchain, how should those interoperate (e.g., with what interfaces) and how many of those should act as validators, something which would help clarify the operational performance and costs, potential issues with scalability and also the robustness and reliability of the technology against security attacks. There are also legal and regulatory challenges in relation to the legal jurisdictions of participant actors. There are economic challenges around who owns and controls the tokens in PoS protocols, who has most of the user accounts and who controls the way that these users access applications and data. There are also organizational challenges around the digital maturity of participant actors, their specific needs, resources and capabilities and how and whether they can negotiate the terms and conditions of their participation.

The key paradox underlying implementations of blockchain technology in healthcare is that the technology needs to have a large number of participants to benefit from scaled decentralized transactions, but at the same time it needs to ensure that all parties are accounted for and trusted, while securing the privacy of their data. Unlike blockchain for cryptocurrencies, blockchain for healthcare needs to have scale with trusted – not anonymous – parties. However, the larger the number of ecosystem participants, the more difficult collective action becomes and the harder it is to define decentralized governance mechanisms.[70]

Notes

1 Lacity, M., Sabherwal, R. and Sørensen, C., 2019. Special issue editorial: delivering business value through enterprise blockchain applications. *MIS Quarterly Executive*, 18(4), p. 11.
2 Manion, S.T. and Bizouati-Kennedy, Y., 2020. *Blockchain for Medical Research: Accelerating Trust in Healthcare*. CRC Press, Boca-raton, USA.
3 Lacity, M., Sabherwal, R. and Sørensen, C., 2019. Special issue editorial: delivering business value through enterprise blockchain applications. *MIS Quarterly Executive*, 18(4), p. 11.
4 Williamson, O.E., 1991. Comparative economic organization: the analysis of discrete structural alternatives. *Administrative Science Quarterly*, 36(2), pp. 269–296; Barthelemy, J., 2003. The seven deadly sins of outsourcing. *Academy of Management Perspectives*, 17(2), pp. 87–98.
5 Lacity, M., Sabherwal, R. and Sørensen, C., 2019. Special issue editorial: delivering business value through enterprise blockchain applications. *MIS Quarterly Executive*, 18(4), p. 11.
6 Nakamoto, S., 2008. Bitcoin: a peer-to-peer electronic cash system. https://bitcoin.org/en/bitcoin-paper.
7 Ibid.
8 Felin, T. and Lakhani, K., 2018. What problems will you solve with blockchain? *MIT Sloan Management Review* 60(1), pp. 32–38; Catalini, C., 2017. How blockchain applications will move beyond finance. *Harvard Business Review*, 2. https://hbsp.harvard.edu/product/H03HRT-PDF-ENG
9 https://pharmaledger.eu/
10 Yuan, Y. and Wang, F.Y., 2018. Blockchain and cryptocurrencies: model, techniques, and applications. *IEEE Transactions on Systems, Man, and Cybernetics: Systems*, 48(9), pp. 1421–1428.
11 See Lamport, L., Shostak, R. and Pease, M., 1982. The Byzantine generals problem. *ACM Transactions on Programming Languages and Systems*, 4(3), pp. 382–401.
12 For example, the Paxos consensus algorithm has been around since the 1990s and is used by Google and Microsoft among others. See Halaburda, H., Sarvary, M. and Haeringer, G., 2022. *Beyond Bitcoin: Economics of Digital Currencies and Blockchain Technologies*. Palgrave Macmillan, 2nd Edition., New York, USA.
13 For an extensive, critical review of mining, see Halaburda, H., Sarvary, M. and Haeringer, G. 2022. *Beyond Bitcoin: Economics of Digital Currencies and Blockchain Technologies*. Palgrave Macmillan, 2nd Edition.
14 Halaburda, H., Sarvary, M. and Haeringer, G., 2022. *Beyond Bitcoin: Economics of Digital Currencies and Blockchain Technologies*. Palgrave Macmillan, 2nd Edition, p. 112.

15 Ibid.

16 Dahabiyeh, L. and Constantinides, P., 2022. Legitimating digital technologies in industry exchange fields: the case of digital signatures. *Information and Organization*, 32(1), p. 100392.

17 Constantinides, P., Henfridsson, O. and Parker, G.G., 2018. Platforms and infrastructures in the digital age. *Information Systems Research*, 29(2), pp. 381–400.

18 Vitalik Buterin, the creator of the Ethereum blockchain infrastructure, proposes three axes of (de) centralization, namely, architectural, political and logical. The political axis is all about control which aligns with the axis proposed in this chapter on governance. The logical axis is about how the architecture – and by extension its governance – splits through interfaces and data structures. It is, thus, a part of the other two axes. See https://medium.com/@VitalikButerin/the-meaning-of-decentralization-a0c92b76a274

19 Chen, H., Pendleton, M., Njilla, L. and Xu, S., 2020. A survey on ethereum systems security: vulnerabilities, attacks, and defenses. *ACM Computing Surveys (CSUR)*, 53(3), pp. 1–43.

20 Often with the off-chain data cryptographically verified through anchoring or oracle-based verifications.

21 Ostrom, E., 1990. *Governing the Commons*. Cambridge, UK: Cambridge University Press; Williamson, O.E., 1996. *The Mechanisms of Governance*. New York, NY: Oxford University Press.

22 De Rossi, L.M., Abbatemarco, N. and Salviotti, G., 2019, January. Towards a Comprehensive Blockchain Architecture Continuum. In *Proceedings of the 52nd Hawaii International Conference on System Sciences.*, University of Hawai'i at Mānoa, Hamilton Library, Honolulu, Hawaii.

23 Beck, R., Müller-Bloch, C. and King, J.L., 2018. Governance in the blockchain economy: A framework and research agenda. *Journal of the Association for Information Systems*, 19(10), p. 1.

24 Buterin, V. 2014. The Ethereum Whitepaper. https://ethereum.org/en/whitepaper/

25 Christidis, K., & Devetsikiotis, M. (2016). Blockchains and smart contracts for the internet of things. *IEEE Access*, 4, pp. 2292–2303; Zhang, Y., Kasahara, S., Shen, Y., Jiang, X. and Wan, J., 2018. Smart contract-based access control for the internet of things. *IEEE Internet of Things Journal*, 6(2), pp. 1594–1605.

26 Beck, R., Müller-Bloch, C. and King, J.L., 2018. Governance in the blockchain economy: A framework and research agenda. *Journal of the Association for Information Systems*, 19(10), p. 1.

27 Halaburda, H., Sarvary, M., and Haeringer, G. 2022. *Beyond Bitcoin: Economics of Digital Currencies and Blockchain Technologies*. Palgrave Macmillan, 2nd Edition, New York, USA

28 See for example the discussion on Ethereum and Ethereum 2.0 https://www.forbes.com/advisor/investing/cryptocurrency/what-is-ethereum-2-merge/

29 Beck, R., Müller-Bloch, C. and King, J.L., 2018. Governance in the blockchain economy: a framework and research agenda. *Journal of the Association for Information Systems*, 19(10), p. 1.

30 Pedersen, A.B., Risius, M. and Beck, R., 2019. A ten-step decision path to determine when to use blockchain technologies. *MIS Quarterly Executive*, 18(2), pp. 99–115.

31 See Deloitte's framework for blockchain implementations in health information exchanges https://www2.deloitte.com/us/en/pages/public-sector/articles/blockchain-opportunities-for-health-care.html

32 https://pharmaledger.eu/

33 PharmaLedger is a Horizon 2020 European project. All project reports and documents are available here: https://pharmaledger.eu/resources-publications/horizon-2020-pharmaledger-grant-agreement-documents/

34 FT investigation into How top health websites are sharing sensitive data with advertisers https://www.ft.com/content/0fbf4d8e-022b-11ea-be59-e49b2a136b8d

35 The European General Data Protection Regulation (GDPR), Article 4, §2 https://gdpr-info.eu/art-4-gdpr/

36 The European General Data Protection Regulation (GDPR), Article 6, §1 https://gdpr-info.eu/art-6-gdpr/

37 The European General Data Protection Regulation (GDPR), Article 4, §11 https://gdpr-info.eu/art-4-gdpr/

38 Guidelines on consent under Regulation 2016/679 (2017) 17/EN WP259, https://ec.europa.eu/newsroom/article29/items/623051

39 The European General Data Protection Regulation (GDPR), Article 4, §2 https://gdpr-info.eu/art-4-gdpr/
40 Ibid.
41 The European General Data Protection Regulation (GDPR), Recital 26, https://gdpr-info.eu/recitals/no-26/
42 https://www.weforum.org/agenda/2021/08/self-sovereign-identity-future-personal-data-ownership/
43 According to the European General Data Protection Regulation (GDPR), Article 5, §1, data ought to be "adequate, relevant and limited to what is necessary in relation to the purposes for which they are processed". What stems from this principle is a requirement to only collect and hold the personal data needed for the specific purpose.
44 https://www.geeksforgeeks.org/zero-knowledge-proof/
45 https://www.clinicaltrialsarena.com/marketdata/featureclinical-trial-patient-recruitment/
46 Fogel, D.B., 2018. Factors associated with clinical trials that fail and opportunities for improving the likelihood of success: a review. *Contemporary Clinical Trials Communications*, 11, pp. 156–164.
47 https://health.ec.europa.eu/system/files/2016-11/annex11_01-2011_en_0.pdf
48 https://www.fda.gov/medical-devices/postmarket-requirements-devices/quality-system-qs-regulationmedical-device-good-manufacturing-practices
49 The OpenDSU Bluepaper is available here: https://docs.google.com/document/d/1CH2Z2DFpEJXDZIUJi6pyS2hh9TxWxhNQlOsAGU8vYZA/edit#heading=h.ua7dqwbjs752
50 Ibid.
51 Yeung, K., 2021. The health care sector's experience of blockchain: a cross-disciplinary investigation of its real transformative potential. *Journal of Medical Internet Research*, 23(12), p. e24109.
52 See for example the CEO of Avaneer Health, a healthcare blockchain technology and services company, discussing possible use cases here https://www.healthcareitnews.com/news/healthcare-blockchain-leader-talks-challenges-and-trends-dlt; also see an opinion piece in *BMC Medicine* where a multidisciplinary group of academics and practitioners discuss the potential of different use cases https://bmcmedicine.biomedcentral.com/articles/10.1186/s12916-019-1296-7
53 https://www.cbo.gov/publication/57126
54 Lu Lundh, A., Lexchin, J., Mintzes, B., Schroll, J.B. and Bero, L., 2017. Industry sponsorship and research outcome. *Cochrane Database of Systematic Reviews*, (2); Goldacre, B., Lane, S., Mahtani, K.R., Heneghan, C., Onakpoya, I., Bushfield, I. and Smeeth, L., 2017. Pharmaceutical companies' policies on access to trial data, results, and methods: audit study. *BMJ*, 358; Weintraub, A. (2016). Why Big Pharma Gets A Failing Grade On Clinical Trial Transparency. Retrieved from https://www.forbes.com/sites/arleneweintraub/2016/08/17/why-big-pharma-gets-a-failing-grade-on-clinical-trial-transparency/#437150406cbd
55 See some recent discussions between economists and regulators here https://www.biopharmadive.com/news/ftc-pharma-mergers-biotech-antitrust-competition/625592/. See a *Financial Times* report on big pharma's $1.4 trillion "deal-making firepower" https://www.ft.com/content/325b75d9-5148-4635-b9c2-63244fa74936
56 Johns Hopkins Bloomberg School of Public Health. Cost of Clinical Trials for New Drug FDA Approval Are Fraction of Total Tab. 2018. https://www.jhsph.edu/news/news-releases/2018/cost-of-clinical-trials-for-new-drug-FDA-approval-are-fraction-of-total-tab.html.
57 Ibid.
58 Mackey, T.K. and Liang, B.A., 2013. Improving global health governance to combat counterfeit medicines: a proposal for a UNODC-WHO-Interpol trilateral mechanism. *BMC Medicine*, 11(1), pp. 1–10.
59 State of Blockchain Adoption on the Pharmaceutical Supply Chain. 2017. IEEE Standards Association. https://blockchain.ieee.org/standards/2017-sba-psc
60 Yli-Huumo, J., Ko, D., Choi, S., Park, S. and Smolander, K., 2016. Where is current research on blockchain technology?—a systematic review. *PloS One*, 11(10), p. e0163477.
61 Kuo, T.T., Kim, H.E. and Ohno-Machado, L., 2017. Blockchain distributed ledger technologies for biomedical and health care applications. *Journal of the American Medical Informatics Association*, 24(6), pp. 1211–1220.

62 Park, Y.R., Lee, E., Na, W., Park, S., Lee, Y. and Lee, J.H., 2019. Is blockchain technology suitable for managing personal health records? Mixed-methods study to test feasibility. *Journal of Medical Internet Research*, 21(2), p. e12533.

63 Ibid.

64 O'Donoghue, O., Vazirani, A.A., Brindley, D. and Meinert, E., 2019. Design choices and trade-offs in health care blockchain implementations: systematic review. *Journal of Medical Internet Research*, 21(5), p. e12426.

65 More data on this here https://www.cnil.fr/sites/default/files/atoms/files/blockchain_en.pdf

66 Park, Y.R., Lee, E., Na, W., Park, S., Lee, Y. and Lee, J.H., 2019. Is blockchain technology suitable for managing personal health records? Mixed-methods study to test feasibility. *Journal of Medical Internet Research*, 21(2), p. e12533.

67 Constantinides, P., 2012. *Perspectives and Implications for the Development of Information Infrastructures*. IGI Global, Hershey, USA; Constantinides, P. and Barrett, M., 2015. Information infrastructure development and governance as collective action. *Information Systems Research*, 26(1), pp. 40–56.

68 I thank James Gannon, VP Quality, Trust & Safety, PharmaLedger Association for this clarification.

69 Gordon, W.J. and Catalini, C., 2018. Blockchain technology for healthcare: facilitating the transition to patient-driven interoperability. *Computational and Structural Biotechnology Journal*, 16, pp. 224–230.

70 One of the most commonly accepted tenets in the literature on collective action is that "the larger the group, the less it will further its common interests" (Olson, 1965, p. 36). Olson, M., 1965. *The Logic of Collective Action: Public Goods and the Theory of Groups*. Cambridge, MA: Harvard University Press; see also Ostrom, E. 1990. *Governing the Commons: The Evolution of Institutions for Collective Action*. Cambridge, MA: Cambridge University Press.

6 Cloud Computing and Federated Learning Infrastructures

Unlike blockchain infrastructures discussed in Chapter 5, an alternative approach to managing data across an ecosystem is data virtualization. Virtualization is a key concept in cloud computing in that it removes all physical infrastructure constraints, enabling users across different geographical locations to use virtual machines for networking, storage, server utilization and deployment of multiple operating systems, applications and data. With virtualization, organizations can manage, maintain and use all the aforementioned components like applications on the web, with the help of cloud service providers. Data virtualization presents unique opportunities to more flexibly governing data across healthcare ecosystems.

In healthcare data can come from electronic patient records, diagnostics and lab tests; they can also come from disease surveillance, immunization records and other registries held at the level of public health agencies; they can come from research into genomics and genetics, as well as clinical trials all of which may reside in biodata banks; but they can also come from an expanding list of data points including mobile apps, wearables and sensors.[1] Given this range of datasets and the computing and data storage requirements they involve, healthcare organizations often have to use multiple different computing resources, often located in different geographical locations. In addition, performing computational analysis of such datasets involves increased computing resources to copy, transfer and download, something that creates more security and regulatory compliance risks, not to mention the costs associated (e.g., cloud egress charges on data downloads). Moreover, the process of copying, transferring and downloading may happen on multiple devices and across operating systems, applications and data formats causing significant bottlenecks.

Data virtualization addresses these issues by providing virtual links to data that may be located in different physical machines. This means that the data never leaves its physical location which preserves security and data integrity. More importantly, data virtualization can perform computational analysis of these virtual data while avoiding compatibility challenges across applications, operating systems and computing configurations. Data virtualization can also leverage the power of federated machine learning technologies that are cloud-based, with cloud providers managing all the hardware, software and server configurations, enabling greater speed and scale for individual organizations. This addresses many of the challenges discussed in relation to blockchain infrastructures, since each organization can have a personalized infrastructure configuration, while keeping control over their own data.

This chapter discusses ways by which healthcare organizations can form ecosystems on federated learning infrastructures. The chapter describes how cloud computing

DOI: 10.4324/9781032619569-8

works, before exploring data virtualization and federated learning infrastructures. It then discusses two use cases of federated learning in healthcare ecosystems: one in medical imaging and one in genomics research. The chapter concludes by discussing the co-innovation and co-adoption challenges of the use of data virtualization in healthcare.

6.1   Cloud Computing, Virtualization and Federated Learning

The scale and speed by which digital technologies are advancing, including the acceleration of data production and consumption, make the technical complexity, operational and financial risks of managing and maintaining a digital infrastructure too high for single healthcare organizations. Chapter 2 has already discussed the technical challenges faced by healthcare organizations, and Chapter 3 has also mapped out the varying levels of digital maturity these organizations experience. Those with high digital maturity tend to operate on cloud computing models, managed by competent technology providers that can orchestrate infrastructures for security, reliability and scale.

Modern technology architectures are built on multiple layers and are modularized, as discussed in Chapter 4. A simplified illustration of the layered modular architecture of digital technology in healthcare is shown in Figure 6.1.

The infrastructure layer is foundational, composed of an operating system, hardware and network components for effective data capture and storage servers as well as curation and interoperability to integrate distributed components that sit on subsequent layers. Built on top of the infrastructure layer is the data analytics and intelligence layer, which captures, processes and analyses data, while deploying machine learning algorithms to

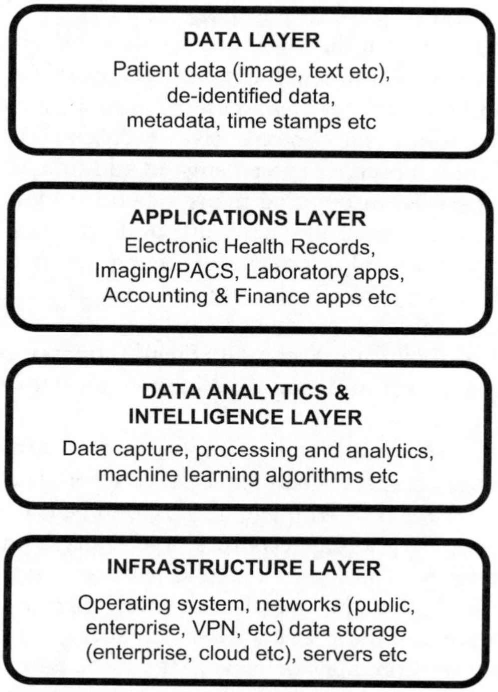

DATA LAYER
Patient data (image, text etc),
de-identified data,
metadata, time stamps etc

APPLICATIONS LAYER
Electronic Health Records,
Imaging/PACS, Laboratory apps,
Accounting & Finance apps etc

**DATA ANALYTICS &
INTELLIGENCE LAYER**
Data capture, processing and analytics,
machine learning algorithms etc

INFRASTRUCTURE LAYER
Operating system, networks (public,
enterprise, VPN, etc) data storage
(enterprise, cloud etc), servers etc

Figure 6.1 The Layered Modular Architecture of Digital Technology in Healthcare.

generate actionable insights. Then, the applications layer includes a number of different applications, from laboratory, radiology, electronic patient records, ward management, accounting and payments, payroll and others, which can be deployed across different devices and information systems. The applications layer is made possible through a set of application programming interfaces (API) that enables different third-party complementors to add value on the ecosystem. Finally, the data layer effectively curates an end-to-end experience for all patients, but also other end-users who use applications on the ecosystem. Components of these layers can be developed by various ecosystem partners and then licensed for use by different users.

6.1.1   Cloud Computing Services and Models

Cloud computing allows this architecture to be virtualized and used on-demand over the Internet on a pay-as-you-go pricing.[2] Instead of buying, owning and maintaining a physical infrastructure and applications, you can access these as a service from cloud providers such as Amazon AWS and Microsoft Azure. Cloud computing removes the cost of expensive physical infrastructures, delivers services at faster computing speeds and higher scale, helps in securing data, apps and infrastructure, provides faster updates to applications and helps manage disaster recovery much more efficiently than on-premises infrastructure.

Cloud computing takes advantage of significant economies of scale in three areas,[3] namely, *supply-side savings,* which essentially refer to large-scale data centers that lower costs per server; *demand-side aggregation,* which refers to the smoothing of overall variability, allowing server utilization rates to increase; and *multitenancy efficiency*, which lowers the application management and server cost per user.

First, supply-side economies of scale emanate from the lower cost of electricity power that large facilities can achieve. While the operators of small data centers must pay the prevailing local rate for electricity, large providers can pay less than the national average rate by locating their data centers in locations with inexpensive electricity supply (including renewable sources) and through bulk purchase agreements. In addition, cloud computing can significantly lower labor costs by automating many repetitive management tasks. This allows technical employees to focus on higher value-add activities like building new capabilities and working through the long queue of user requests every digital unit contends with. Further, large commercial cloud providers such as Amazon AWS and Microsoft Azure are often better able to bring deep expertise to address security and reliability needs than a typical digital services unit. Finally, operators of large cloud data centers have better buying power and can get discounts on hardware purchases of up to 30 percent over smaller buyers.

Second, while supply-side economies of scale depend on the overall cost of technology investment, demand-side aggregation depends on costs of actually utilized resources such as computing, network and storage. A key economic advantage of the cloud is its ability to address variability in resource utilization. By pooling resources, variability is diversified away, balancing out utilization patterns. The larger the pool of resources, the smoother the aggregate demand profile, the higher the overall utilization rate and the cheaper and more efficiently the organization can meet its end-user demands.

Third, there is another important source of economies of scale that can be harnessed only if the application is written as a multitenant application. That is, rather than running an application instance for each customer – as is done for on-premises applications and most hosted applications – in a multitenant application, multiple customers use a single instance of the application simultaneously, as in the case of Microsoft 365, that also includes a Copilot, a corporate version of GPT-4 (more on this in Chapter 7). This has two important economic benefits. First, in a single-tenant instance, each customer has to pay for its own application management. In a multitenant instance such as Microsoft 365, that cost is shared across a large set of customers, driving application labor costs per customer toward zero. This can result in a meaningful reduction in overall cost, especially for complex applications. Second, by moving to a multitenant model with a single instance, server overhead can be spread across all customers. Applications can be entirely multitenant by being completely written to take advantage of these benefits or can achieve partial multitenancy by leveraging shared services provided by the cloud platform. The greater the use of such shared services, the greater the application will benefit from these multitenancy economies of scale.

Capturing benefits from supply-side economies of scale in server capacity, demand-side aggregation of workloads and the multitenant application model is not a straightforward task with today's technology. For instance, multitenancy and demand-side aggregation is often difficult for developers or even sophisticated digital units to implement on their own. If not done correctly, it could end up either significantly raising the costs of developing applications (thus at least partially nullifying the increased budget room for new app development) or capturing only a small subset of the savings previously described. It all depends on the type of applications being considered for outsourcing on the cloud, as shown in Figure 6.2.

First, an on-premises technology infrastructure presents the biggest level of responsibility to individual healthcare organizations since they act both as a user and an owner-manager. This means that organizations are responsible for maintaining, updating and replacing components across all layers, as and when needed, including handling security and disaster recovery.

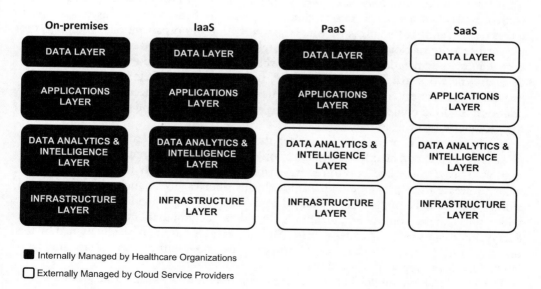

Figure 6.2 Types of Cloud Services.

Second, infrastructure-as-a-service (IaaS) is the first step away from on-premises infrastructure. Individual organizations can outsource to a third-party provider infrastructure services such as storage and virtualization. Organizations are responsible for providing the operating system, applications and data and analytics, while a third-party provider manages the network, servers, virtualization and storage needs. Individual organizations do not have to maintain or update their own data centers. They access and control the infrastructure via an API provided by the third-party provider. This gives flexibility to purchase only the components an organizations needs and can scale those up or down as needed. The main challenges with IaaS are security and service reliability issues due to multitenant systems, where the third-party provider must share infrastructure resources with multiple organizations.

Platform-as-a-service (PaaS) is a service model where a third-party provider hosts the hardware and software and delivers this as an integrated platform to individual organizations. PaaS offers shared services, advanced management and automation features that allow developers to focus directly on application logic rather than on engineering their application to scale. PaaS enabled developers to use built-in software components to create their applications, which cuts down the amount of code they have to write themselves.

Software-as-a-service (SaaS) is the most comprehensive form of cloud computing services, with third-party providers delivering an entire solution to individual organizations across all layers of the technology architecture. Software updates, bug fixes and general software maintenance are handled by the third-party provider, and individual organizations access all applications and data via a web dashboard or API. There is no installation of the software on individual machines and organization-wide and group-wide access is smoother, more reliable and secure.

There are three types of cloud computing models to deploy SaaS, PaaS and IaaS, namely, public cloud, private cloud and hybrid cloud.[4] In a public cloud model, the cloud service providers retain ownership and operate all the hardware, software and other infrastructure components. A web browser can be used to access these services and control individual accounts. Public clouds provide the benefit of increased scale at a lower cost given that the infrastructure is shared with other organizations. Although the physical security of cloud providers is unmatched, there is a shared responsibility model that requires organizations to subscribe to those cloud services to ensure their applications and network are secure, for example, by monitoring packets for malware or by providing encryption of data at rest and in motion.[5] Most concerns raised with the adoption of cloud computing relate to the risks of public cloud models in compromising the safety and security of data.[6]

In contrast, in a private cloud model the cloud computing resources are placed physically on-site at a healthcare organization's premises. Digitally mature organizations that have heavily invested in on-premises infrastructure frequently leverage that investment to create their private cloud. Although this offers a big financial benefit, private clouds must still be supported, managed and eventually upgraded or replaced, all of which falls squarely on the organization's shoulders, including adding physical security, encryption to network and cybersecurity. Since private clouds are typically owned by the organization, there is no sharing of infrastructure, no multitenancy issues and zero latency for local applications and users.

The hybrid cloud model benefits from a combination of public and private cloud computing resources. A hybrid cloud can deliver better flexibility and agility, including optimization benefits in achieving security and compliance across applications and services. Finally, many digitally mature organizations have multicloud deployments with different cloud service providers to mitigate risks of exposure and benefit from different configurations and services.[7]

6.1.2 *Virtualization*

Cloud computing builds on virtualization technology. Indeed, cloud computing is but one type of virtualization. Other types[8] include desktop or *operating system virtualization*, where a user can use multiple operating systems on a single computer Windows, Linux, MacOS); *network virtualization*, where physical networks are combined into a virtual network allowing system administrators to group devices and restrict access to others outside the group; *storage virtualization*, where a group of physical storage devices are combined in a virtual storage network allowing applications and servers to access information from storage systems without needing to know which physical or virtual device the data is stored on; *application virtualization*, where an application is stored virtually on a server and then accessed by the user's device through the server, instead of being installed directly on the device; and *data virtualization*, where users can access data without needing to know exactly where the data is stored or what format it is in. Data is aggregated without moving or changing the original data, so it can be quickly accessed from any device.

As shown in Figure 6.3, the whole technology architecture can be virtualized and this is an instance of SaaS, as described in the previous section and Figure 6.2. Depending on the needs of each organization, different layers and modules of the architecture may remain on-premises and physically managed on site, whereas others can be managed virtually as virtual machines.

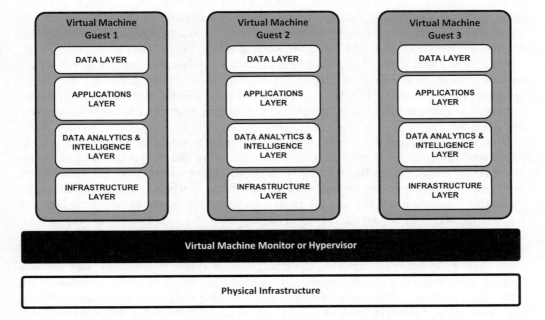

Figure 6.3 A Virtual Machine Monitor.

A virtual machine monitor or hypervisor is a layer of software that sits between a virtual machine and the physical infrastructure.[9] A hypervisor abstracts operating systems, applications and data from their underlying hardware. The physical hardware that a hypervisor runs on is typically referred to as a host machine, whereas the virtual machines the hypervisor creates and supports are collectively called guest machines.

There are two types of hypervisors: Type 1 and Type 2 hypervisors. Both hypervisor types can virtualize computing resources, but based on their location in the architecture, each type virtualizes these resources differently. Type 1 hypervisors[10] run directly on the host machine's physical infrastructure, and they are referred to as bare-metal hypervisors.[11] Type 1 hypervisors do not have to load an underlying operating system; they are, thus, more efficient and secure. This is because each guest virtual machine has its own operating system, something that ensures an attack is logically isolated and cannot spread to others running on the same hardware. Type 1 hypervisors can scale to virtualize higher workloads across computing resources. In addition, Type 1 hypervisors often provide support for software-defined storage and networking, which creates additional security and portability for virtualized workloads. However, such features come with much higher costs and greater contract requirements.

Type 2 hypervisors,[12] by contrast, are installed on top of an existing operating system and that is why they are referred to as hosted hypervisors. Although Type 1 and Type 2 hypervisors can provide the same virtualization functionality, by being hosted, Type 2 hypervisors suffer from unavoidable latency. Also, any security flaws or vulnerabilities in the host operating system can potentially compromise all of the virtual machines running above it. Consequently, Type 2 hypervisors are generally not used for data center computing and are reserved for client or end-user systems where performance and security are lesser concerns. They also come at a lower cost than Type 1 hypervisors and make an ideal test platform compared to production virtualized environments or the cloud. For example, software developers might use a Type 2 hypervisor to create virtual machines upon which they can test a software product prior to release.

Both Type 1 and Type 2 hypervisors use hardware acceleration technologies,[13] which perform many of the process-intensive tasks needed to create and manage virtual resources on a computer. Hardware acceleration improves the virtualization performance and the number of virtual machines a computer can host above what the hypervisor can do alone.

Virtualization has all the benefits already mentioned in relation to cloud computing. More specifically, in relation to the growth of data in healthcare and the need for better governance, virtualization has the ability to consolidate multiple physical data servers into a single server that can run many virtual machines, enabling a much higher rate of utilization. This reduces the overall power and cooling requirements, including the necessity to add to or construct additional data centers. By extension, with fewer servers, virtualization reduces hardware maintenance costs and the time system administrators take to perform many other routine tasks.[14]

Virtualization benefits from, on the one hand, resource distribution among users located in different physical locations and, on the other hand, resource isolation, since virtualization components – whether those are operating systems, applications or data – are self-contained virtual machines that operate in an isolated virtual environment. This virtual environment not only secures sensitive data but also allows distributed users to remain connected.

6.1.3   *Federated Learning*

Cloud computing and data virtualization offer opportunities to scale resources and capabilities across multiple healthcare organizations that are part of the same ecosystem. Healthcare organizations can benefit from federated learning, a type of machine learning (ML) that enables a group of organizations, or groups within the same organization, to collaboratively and iteratively train a shared ML model. In federated learning, no data is shared outside individual organizations or groups within the same organization. The federated infrastructure can be made up of diverse configurations, such as geographic regions and timezones, or across groups within the same organization. Federated learning enables the implementation of ML in use cases where it is generally difficult to share data between organizations due to privacy, regulatory or technical constraints, such as, for example, clinical trials, as discussed in Chapter 5.

Another use case is the use of genomic and other biodata across private and public sector organizations to develop novel, more efficient diagnostics and therapies for rare and chronic diseases and to better monitor and improve existing therapies.[15] In recent years, there have been many initiatives to establish digital platform ecosystems to maximize the use of genomic and other biodata. For example, the Human Genome Project, the HapMap project and the ICGC/TCGA Pan-Cancer Analysis of Whole Genomes Consortium are great examples of platform ecosystem-based genomics projects.[16] More recently, the European COVID-19 Data Platform, a joint initiative by the European Commission, the European Bioinformatics Institute of the European Molecular Biology Laboratory (EMBL-EBI), the Elixir infrastructure and the COMPARE project, seeks to investigate the genetic determinants of COVID-19 susceptibility, severity and outcomes. These and other such initiatives take advantage of cloud computing and federated learning, as reported in a recent OECD report.[17]

To understand the process of implementing federated learning, it is important to clarify some high-level concepts of ML. ML uses mathematical algorithms to analyze patterns in data and the relationships between them. In contrast to rule-based software programming, ML algorithms learn from data to discover their own rules and can improve their performance with experience. ML algorithms are deployed in artificial neural networks across multiple layers. By adding more layers and more units of data within each layer, an artificial neural network gains more "depth" and can represent functions of increasing complexity.[18] A deep neural network consists of multiple artificial *neurons* that take input from data with corresponding weights and then a ML algorithm performs a function before producing an output, as shown in Figure 6.4.

Artificial neural networks are collections of neurons that are connected such that the outputs of some neurons can become inputs to other neurons. Artificial neural networks learn to map a series of inputs from different types of biodata (e.g., genomic, proteomic, epigenomic, metabolomic) to an output (e.g., the probability that the data can point to several clinical categories). Every layer transforms one set of outputs to another through different ML algorithm functions until objects of interest can be detected (e.g., a genetic determinant of COVID-19).[19]

ML models (i.e., ML algorithms plus the artificial neural networks within which they are deployed) require large datasets before they can learn to perform autonomously. The key problem is that, unlike other sectors – for example retail – that have an abundance of datasets with which to train their ML models, in healthcare such datasets are limited and often subject to ethical approval. For example, unlike imaging datasets

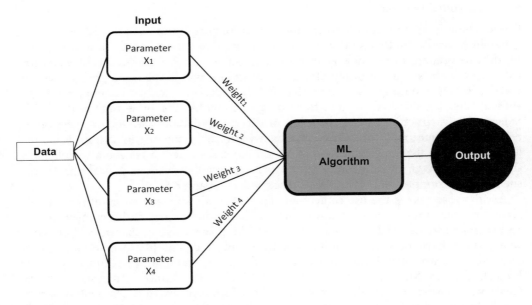

Figure 6.4 An Artificial Neuron.

used for non-clinical tasks that are publicly available such as the ImageNet database, which contains more than 14 million clearly annotated images,[20] medical image analysis most often depends on private datasets that are limited. Private datasets, usually held by private or national payers and big hospitals or other healthcare providers, require data preparation including manual labeling and annotation that is time consuming and prone to errors.[21] Errors can be made on the basis of individual diseases and the patient's medical history, but can also be made on the basis of inclination or prejudice for or against someone or something.[22] For example, one study[23] showed that one can have eight different findings on a chest X-ray, many of which have overlapping features and can be difficult to use for diagnosis. Such errors can make it into the training sample used for ML models subjecting their performance to conflicting outcomes. Indeed, ML models trained on a single dataset from a single healthcare organization may easily overfit data on cases that are most prevalent in that organization, resulting in a strong bias. For example, datasets containing only one modality may bias ML models toward that modality, capturing irrelevant data as significant predictors.[24] Also, the quality of a single organization's dataset will vary based on the number of patients, type or number of diagnostic and other devices that integrate with AI workflow systems, and the number of experts available at that organization. This can, once again, generate errors in ML model outcomes.

ML models require clearly annotated data upon which they can be trained prior to being implemented in different applications such as diagnostics, treatment predictions, gene sequencing and drug development. Data annotation is part of the training process which involves giving labels and metadata tags to different types of data. Data annotations establish the "ground truth" for ML models. "Ground truth refers to the actual nature of the problem that is the target of a machine learning model, reflected by the relevant datasets associated with the use case in question".[25] Ground truth is set by human experts and refers to the accuracy of the input data to train a ML model to achieve desired outputs. Depending on the complexity of the problem, ML models may require more datasets, depicting normal, abnormal and "edge cases", that is, rare cases. The key problem is that it is very difficult to get data on rare cases. For example, in a breast cancer screening population, only about 7 out of 1,000 mammograms actually have cancer. Getting training data from normal samples will often be much easier.[26] This means many rare samples are, almost by definition, not included in the training set. Rare samples can deviate so much from the data distribution that they end up in areas of the feature space for which the ML model has not been optimized to detect. This lack of training data can have a significant impact of the performance of ML models and the detection of disease.

In federated learning, these data problems are mitigated to a great degree given that participating organizations share insights from their data to collaboratively train a global ML model, improving on it iteratively. This happens without actually sharing data between organizations; rather virtual links to the data are created instead, as explained earlier. Each of these participating organizations may submit insights from heterogeneous datasets with different parameters, features and sizes. Organizations download the global ML model from the cloud, usually a pre-trained foundation model. Foundation models are trained on a broad set of unlabeled data that can be used for different tasks.[27] Then individual participating organizations can train this foundation model on their private data, using their own data annotations and labels and local weights. Each participating organization then sends their local model updates back to the cloud. Iteration after iteration, the federated training continues until the model is fully trained, while normalizing local biases and errors.[28] The process is illustrated in Figure 6.5.

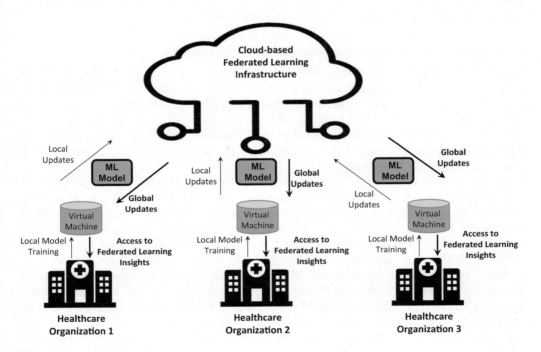

Figure 6.5 Federated Learning.

Federated learning can be implemented along different ecosystem models, including a *centralized model*, where an ecosystem orchestrator coordinates the computing resources, while a set of participant organizations provide distinct data and contribute to the training process; a *decentralized model* whereby there is no central orchestrator but rather all participant organizations share coordination responsibilities as a consortium; and finally a *heterogeneous model* which is a hybrid of the centralized and decentralized models.[29] These models reflect the architecture configurations discussed in Chapter 4. The orchestrator or consortium of orchestrators determines the responsibilities of all participant organizations, including the design and implementation of the global ML model, the federated learning rounds (e.g., training iterations, configuration of the model, adding/editing and removing data labels and annotations, and validation) and the privacy, security and regulatory requirements of accessing and using the data.

6.2   Use Cases of Federated Learning in Healthcare Ecosystems

As discussed in the previous section, there are currently both public and private sector initiatives, as well as combinations of those, where different organizations are developing digital platform ecosystems to leverage federated learning capabilities.[30] The next two subsections provide two use cases of federated learning in healthcare ecosystems. The first one examines the use of federated learning in a large-scale study across 20 healthcare organizations in five continents that used chest X-ray imaging data in addition to clinical data to determine hospital triage for level of care and oxygen requirement in patients with COVID-19. The second use case examines the use of federated learning in genomics research, by leveraging data across two healthcare organizations in the UK with the help of a commercial federated learning platform.

6.2.1   Use Case 1: Federated Learning in Medical Imaging Analysis

Chapter 1 has provided an extensive discussion of the devastation brought by the COVID-19 pandemic across different healthcare ecosystems. At the same time, the COVID-19 pandemic has fueled large-scale experimentation of emergent technologies and distributed datasets that would not have been possible under different circumstances. In particular, the COVID-19 pandemic provided incentives for federated data sharing and model training and testing, while circumventing the usual ethical hurdles of research and development in healthcare.[31]

One such large-scale study[32] was spearheaded by Mass General Brigham (MGB), a Boston-based non-profit hospital and physician network that includes Brigham and Women's Hospital and Massachusetts General Hospital. MGB developed a foundational ML model with inputs from chest X-ray images, vital signs, demographic data and laboratory values. The output of the foundational ML model was predictive risk scores for COVID-19 severe outcomes[33] that could aid in triaging patients by clinicians.

Based on the MGB foundational ML model, 20 healthcare organizations spread around the world, including North and South America, Europe and Asia, developed a federated learning model called EXAM (electronic medical record (EMR) chest X-ray AI model) deployed across a 34-layer convolutional neural network. Ground truth was assigned based on patient oxygen therapy after 24 and 72-hour periods from initial admission to emergency care. The EXAM model was trained using a cohort of 16,148 cases across the 20 healthcare organizations, with local updates and global federated learning insights being fed in each participating organization.

As the study reports, "Local models that were trained using unbalanced cohorts (for example, mostly mild cases of COVID-19) markedly benefited from the FL approach, with a substantial improvement in prediction average AUC performance for categories with only a few cases". In addition, "In the case of client sites with relatively small datasets, the best FL model markedly outperformed not only the local model but also those trained on larger datasets from five client sites".[34]

Overall, "EXAM achieved an average area under the curve (AUC) >0.92 for predicting outcomes at 24 and 72 hours from the time of initial presentation to the emergency room, and it provided 16% improvement in average AUC measured across all participating sites and an average increase in generalizability of 38% when compared with models trained at a single site using that site's data". In addition, in relation to predicting "mechanical ventilation treatment or death at 24 hours at the largest independent test site, EXAM achieved a sensitivity of 0.950 and specificity of 0.882".[35]

This was one of the first applications of federated learning in medical imaging at a global scale to address global epidemics. It provides a proof of concept for an ecosystem-wide collaboration in the use of AI technologies and distributed data governance and analysis. It provides evidence on how federated ML models can capture more diversity than locally trained ML models, while mitigating errors and biases in the data.

6.2.2 Use Case 2: Federated Learning in Genomics Research

A second use case comes from the field of genomics research. In the UK, Lifebit[36] is pioneering the use of federated learning in genomics research by providing a patented[37] PaaS platform. The Lifebit platform ensures that no data leaves the Trusted Research Environment (TRE) of data custodians, i.e., participating organizations who own the data. According to the UK Health Data Research Alliance, a TRE is a "Data Safe Haven" or "Secure Data Environment" that (emphasis in original), *"operates as a safe setting that approved researchers (Safe people) can only access via a virtual desktop interface (VDI). Only de-identified data is accessible by researchers (Safe data). Research is overseen by a review of projects (Safe projects) involving participants, with publicly accessible lay summaries providing transparency. Only summary data can be exported from the TRE through an Airlock and only after manual review (Safe output)"*.[38] The Five Safes framework is being increasingly adopted by data platform providers, including the UK's National Institute for Health Data Research,[39] OpenSafely[40] and Genomics England.[41]

Lifebit implements the Five Safes framework by providing an integrated system of internal controls, automated processes, monitoring and risk assessment to establish a highly robust and secure end-to-end platform. In addition, within the data custodian's TRE, data is transformed into standardized formats such as the OMOP common data model,[42] via automated Extract, Transform, Load (ETL) pipelines.[43] Following data transformation and de-identification, data is stored in a data repository within the data custodian's TRE, where it is made available to approved researchers. Within each data custodian's TRE, verified administrators can specify permissions to data repositories, workflow systems and cloud computing resources on a per-user and per-workspace basis via role-based access control. The Lifebit platform enables integration with third-party authentication systems (e.g., Okta,[44] AuthO[45]), something which allows participating organizations to maintain their privacy protection processes.

Data custodians retain full security over their data at all times and only analysis and computation are taken to external datasets and cohorts via APIs. At the same time, Lifebit enables users to segregate genomic and clinical data types within the platform, while helping them to meet compliance requirements such as GDPR, and security requirements such as ISO 27001, but also standards such as those of GA4GH.[46] Data is encrypted in storage, in transfer and during analysis.[47] Data can only be de-encrypted by authenticated staff, and the security network imposes additional constraints on which specific users can access, view or edit encrypted files. Further, data does not persist beyond purposes directly relevant to the research. By default, Lifebit's platform is configured not to allow data to be exported or downloaded out of a data custodian's TRE and while integrating with a participating organization's data export controls. For example, with Genomics England, Lifebit has taken an integration approach, enabling authorized users to export approved, aggregate-level data using Genomics England's Airlock process.[48] This feature enables authorized personnel to approve and validate the purpose of any data download.

Lifebit's federated platform provides an open ecosystem that is technology and vendor agnostic, enabling participating organizations to customize their TRE with additional third-party applications, tools and data via open API.[49] Lifebit's platform offers a "private-by-default" design of data access, whereby no party has a complete view of the entire dataset and where participating organizations have access to highly reliable, secure and scalable infrastructure.

The Lifebit platform has been applied in a DARE UK (Data and Analytics Research Environments UK) project. DARE UK is a program funded by UK Research and Innovation (UKRI) "to design and deliver coordinated and trustworthy national data research infrastructure to support cross-domain research for public good".[50] As part of this program, Lifebit provided its platform to enable federated analysis between two TREs, namely, a "patient-centred dataset" in the TRE of Genomics England and a "discovery research dataset" in the TRE of the University of Cambridge's Biomedical Research Centre called CYNAPSE (in partnership with Cambridge University Hospitals NHS Foundation Trust). The use case aimed at demonstrating privacy preservation across both datasets, without disclosing potentially re-identifiable patient information from one TRE to researchers in the other.

The use case combined data from both TRE on normal and tumor whole genome sequence samples of cancer patients to explore somatic mutational signatures. Several requirements were met including the successful implementation of GA4GH standards, parallel analyses performed within the TRE of Genomics England and the University of Cambridge, followed by a federated analysis, and exporting of aggregated results (non-identifiable summary statistics) via the Airlock process (i.e., with no risk of re-identification). This federated learning enabled a more scalable, automated and continuous process than the current manual design, while avoiding the significant costs and risk of data leaks associated with moving large datasets between TRE. The use case has also achieved engagement with patients and the public about the concept of federation, demonstrating a methodology that strengthens the safety of patient data. The use case has demonstrated how federated learning can help contribute to reducing the gap between discovery research and clinical translation, through analysis and immediate validation across data cohorts.

Despite these benefits, this use case was only a proof-of-concept study and several challenges remain. A number of learning points were reported as ways of pushing forward the federation of large-scale genomic data infrastructures.[51] These learning points are discussed in the next section, while highlighting key co-innovation and co-adoption challenges for federated learning platform ecosystems.

6.3   Co-Innovation and Co-Adoption Challenges

To start with, achieving a federation partnership between data custodians and data consumers such as researchers is not trivial requiring collective agreements over joint value propositions, co-innovation and co-adoption plans, as discussed in Chapter 4. Even for two data custodians as in the second use case discussed above, the incentives and value capture opportunities have to outweigh the risks. Establishing such incentives becomes even more challenging in cases where there are multiple data custodians from multiple geographical locations as in use case 1. COVID-19 created the necessary conditions and incentives for use case 1 to materialize, but under normal circumstances, such large-scale collaboration may present significant challenges.

Ecosystem actors have to agree on what each partner brings to the ecosystem and what they can expect to receive from others. For example, in the second use case, Genomics England provided more than 130,000 whole genomes derived from de-identified NHS patient-centered data, while the University of Cambridge (CYNAPSE) provided a disparate collection of de-identified and anonymized datasets representing a wide array of discovery research datasets. The data in these two TREs were not amenable to pooling; they were both too large to move and could not be physically pooled for legal, regulatory and practical reasons.[52] Yet both partners benefitted from the collaboration with each other because the discovery and validation opportunities offered by combining subsets of data from the two TREs were significant. The ability to increase the power for discovery and the potential for seeking validation in NHS patient cohorts was immediate. Finally, Lifebit brought their unique platform to enable federated learning to take place between the two TRE. Lifebit provided the right levels of security, while ensuring compliance with industry-wide standards and while offering open-source tools and interfaces to enable third-party integration.

The key difference from other types of ecosystem collaborations is that, for the benefits of federated learning to be realized, data custodians together with the platform orchestrator (e.g., a consortium of organizations in use case 1 – a decentralized model; Lifebit in use case 2 – a centralized model) have to engage in multiple rounds of review and assessment to guarantee that data governance expectations for each data custodian are adhered to. The more complex and heterogeneous the datasets held by each data custodian and the more diverse the data projects that researchers engage in, the higher the number and the more sensitive the data governance expectations will be. Each data custodian would expect to receive a data protection impact assessment (DPIA), at every federated learning update. Such DPIA would provide a risk assessment with evidence of continued improvement of each dataset's security, while also providing a plan to address vulnerabilities in the longer term. This process may be time consuming, but paramount to ensuring the sustainability of the federated platform ecosystem. In addition, using a common data model aligned with FAIR data principles focusing on activities that enable data to be findable, accessible, interoperable and reusable[53] across participating organizations would also ensure best practices. Data standardization and governance need to be clearly defined upfront and communicated to all participating organizations, including data custodians and data consumers.

In addition to challenges to data governance as experienced between participating organizations, there are challenges to data and ML model manipulation from malicious attacks outside the ecosystem. An attacker can access and manipulate a local ML model of one of the participating organizations, resulting in a malicious update in the global ML model. Further, if messages between the central server and a local device are intercepted, a malicious attacker can access the data in the local device by means of some emerging techniques such as model inversion of the model updates,[54] gradient inversion,[55] inference attacks,[56] backdoor attacks,[57] Sybil attacks[58] and adversarial attacks.[59] The more organizations participate in the federated learning platform and the more diverse their architecture configurations and security policies, the more opportunities are provided for such attacks. Security strategies that mitigate these risks include advanced encryption of model submissions, secure authentication of all parties, traceability of actions, differential privacy, verification systems, execution integrity, model confidentiality and protection against adversarial attacks.[60] Use case 1 discussed earlier used many of these security strategies successfully to avoid some of the aforementioned attacks.[61]

Beyond these security challenges, federated learning platforms generate translational outcomes that include not only new diagnostics and therapies but also changes to existing approaches to treatment, better risk stratification and preventive medicine.[62] As such, federated learning platform ecosystems operate with different economies of value than other innovation ecosystems, involving not just financial investments and technological value propositions, but also input data that get translated into new knowledge outputs built on synergistic combinations of resources and capabilities. Such ecosystems involve varied actors across the range of research – the public and patients, clinical and research staff, commercial actors such as pharmaceutical and insurance companies, funders, government and policymakers. However, each of these actors has different conceptions of value. A commercial actor will be seeking to commercialize knowledge, while patients and the public will be seeking social and health value from the knowledge outputs. Awareness of the value conceptions of different ecosystem actors is important as it can help produce mutually agreeable business models.[63]

Federated learning platform ecosystems in genomics in particular manage data that is largely contributed by, and that concern, the public, including patients and research participants. As a result, such ecosystems depend on the involvement of the public as integral partners in the research. Moreover, public funding also underpins much of the research generating and analyzing this data, and many of the platform providers themselves, as in the case of Lifebit. This public involvement points to the production of a common good such as improved prediction, diagnostics, and treatment of emergent and known diseases. This implies that each ecosystem actor has not only rights that must be respected but also that each owes each other responsibilities toward the common good.[64] By reciprocating rights and obligations, the platform ecosystem can operate fairly and effectively for a mutually beneficial value toward such a common good.

The promise of a common good via federated learning platform ecosystems can only be realized if trust is achieved.[65] Trust is instrumental in increasing research participation and improving the perception of research by the public.[66] Trust can only be achieved if ecosystem actors address the concerns about potential harm, and inform research with cultural and individual patient values and expectations into oversight and governance structures.[67] Issues of data security, privacy and commercial access to data also have important implications for achieving public trust.[68] Protection of privacy, data security and a clear and transparent governance framework are key in this respect. Data sharing and research collaboration may not be a barrier to public trust provided that privacy is protected, there is sufficient ethical oversight and data custodians are shown to successfully contribute to the common good.

Despite the promise of a common good, however, collaborations with commercial organizations, especially ones that reside in other countries, remain problematic for some participants. Commercial involvement in research, and the idea that genomics and biodata resources can be monetized, is one of the most problematic aspects of cross-sector collaboration in terms of achieving trust.[69] Value sharing, especially giving health benefits back to the biobank, donor or community, could possibly help remedy any erosion in trust associated with these concerns but such value sharing is difficult to implement in practice.[70] There is therefore a need to support ongoing discussions about the role of research partnerships between public and private sectors, while involving patient and public representatives in such discussions. Participant engagement underpins trust in the research and helps to maintain levels of participation in the research, as well as improve its relevance and utility.

Beyond public engagement and trust building, federated learning platforms are also subject to intellectual property (IP) rights contests in relation to genomic inventions.[71] Because of the length of the development and regulatory process, IP rights are integral to the translation of research into clinically relevant outcomes in health innovation. IP frameworks become increasingly important as research projects develop and outputs mature. However, beyond the controversy around gene sequence patents in current and future genomics research, IP is likely to arise on a much broader range of innovations including the development of ML algorithms and artificial neural networks. Still, there is ongoing legal uncertainty in relation to the ownership and protection of biotechnology-related products.[72] The initial allocation of ownership depends to some extent on the terms of the IP legislation and case law of the jurisdiction in which the invention or creation first arises. The allocation of IP rights is also highly dependent on the terms of the contracts and research agreements through which access to the federated learning platform is granted. Further, issues around the allocation and licensing of IP rights on downstream innovations implicate questions on trust discussed above. The existence of these IP rights, allocation of ownership and the manner of their exploitation can unsettle expectations as ethical concerns about the role of IP in genomics translational research remain.[73] Failures of transparency and the lack of public discussion have the potential to impact public trust and ultimately the sustainability of the platform.

The extent to which ecosystem orchestrators wish to exercise control over IP varies. In most cases, it may be practical and desirable that those accessing the platform would own their own IP, as they are in the best place to develop it appropriately. For example, some federated learning platforms, such as GA4GH, make their IP open source so that it can be freely used and adapted for the common good. At the same time, federated learning platforms should be cautious about employing open-source licenses, if controlled access, fees for service, commercial secrecy and patenting will ultimately be employed, because to do so risks undermining trust, as discussed earlier. Moreover, notions of openness are relatively unhelpful when platforms move beyond mere access to data to questions of ownership of the innovation developed from that data, where there is unlikely to be any intention or attempt to develop innovative products on an open basis.

Other attempts to formulate licenses for genomic IP and to seek to harmonize high-level policies and practices include initiatives such as patent pools and clearinghouses.[74] Some high-profile initiatives of this nature exist in relation to COVID-19 such as the COVID-19 Technology Access Pool (C-TAP) spearheaded by the World Health Organization.[75] On the other hand, exclusive licences risk foreclosing further research and development of whole areas of technological development. Exclusive licences may give rise to problematic monopolies and IP guidelines and policies, therefore caution against such licences unless unavoidable.[76]

Federated learning platforms have great potential to use innovative means of governing licences and IP rights to both advance innovation and the public interest. Additionally, and importantly, federated learning platforms are also well placed to assess and monitor the impact of their policies on downstream access and availability. Moreover, as the gatekeeper to information, they have sufficient bargaining power to implement these principles – and they have the imperative to do so, to safeguard the participants, and further develop and advance existing governance frameworks.

Evidently, many of the governance challenges for federated learning platforms are similar to the challenges that have been discussed in Chapters 4 and 5. Ecosystem-wide governance of the risks associated with co-innovation and co-adoption is key to the successful operation of federated learning platforms and can be an effective means to address the challenges and realize the opportunities in novel therapies, vaccines and diagnostics.

Notes

1 Lauer, K.B., Smith, A., Blomberg, N., Sitjà, X.P., Talbot-Cooper, C., Rothe, H. and Conde, D.S., 2021. Open data: a driving force for innovation in the life sciences. *F1000Research*, 10(828), p. 828.

2 Weinhardt, C., Anandasivam, A., Blau, B., Borissov, N., Meinl, T., Michalk, W. and Stößer, J., 2009. Cloud computing – a classification, business models, and research directions. *Business & Information Systems Engineering*, 1, pp. 391–399; Al-Roomi, M., Al-Ebrahim, S., Buqrais, S. and Ahmad, I., 2013. Cloud computing pricing models: a survey. *International Journal of Grid and Distributed Computing*, 6(5), pp. 93–106.

3 Boss G., Malladi P., Quan S., Legregni L. and Hall H., 2007. Cloud computing. Technical Report, IBM high performance on demand solutions, 2007-10-08, Version 1.0.

4 Fehling, C., Leymann, F., Retter, R., Schupeck, W. and Arbitter, P., 2014. *Cloud Computing Patterns: Fundamentals to Design, Build, and Manage Cloud Applications* (Vol. 545). Berlin: Springer.

5 Subashini, S. and Kavitha, V., 2011. A survey on security issues in service delivery models of cloud computing. *Journal of Network and Computer Applications*, 34(1), pp. 1–11.

6 Griebel, L., Prokosch, H.U., Köpcke, F., Toddenroth, D., Christoph, J., Leb, I., Engel, I. and Sedlmayr, M., 2015. A scoping review of cloud computing in healthcare. *BMC Medical Informatics and Decision Making*, 15(1), pp. 1–16; Chenthara, S., Ahmed, K., Wang, H. and Whittaker, F., 2019. Security and privacy-preserving challenges of e-health solutions in cloud computing. *IEEE Access*, 7, pp. 74361–74382.

7 Mosco, V., 2015. *To the Cloud: Big Data in a Turbulent World*. Routledge.

8 See https://aws.amazon.com/what-is/virtualization/

9 Portnoy, M., 2012. *Virtualization Essentials*. John Wiley & Sons.

10 Some well-known Type 1 hypervisors include VMware vSphere; Microsoft Hyper-V; KVM, an open source virtualization architecture made for Linux distributions, Xen hypervisor, another open source technology; Oracle VM; and Citrix Hypervisor.

11 See https://aws.amazon.com/what-is/virtualization/

12 Some well-known Type 2 hypervisors include Oracle VM VirtualBox; VMware Workstation Pro and VMware Fusion; QEMU, an open source virtualization technology; and Parallels Desktop, primarily geared toward macOS admins.

13 See for example https://learn.microsoft.com/en-us/xamarin/android/get-started/installation/android-emulator/hardware-acceleration?pivots=macos

14 Portnoy, M., 2012. *Virtualization Essentials*. John Wiley & Sons, Indianapolis, USA.

15 Garden, H., Hawkins, N., and Winickoff, D., 2021. Building and sustaining collaborative platforms in genomics and biobanks for health innovation, *OECD Science, Technology and Industry Policy Papers*, No. 102, OECD Publishing, Paris. https://www.oecd-ilibrary.org/science-and-technology/building-and-sustaining-collaborative-platforms-in-genomics-and-biobanks-for-health-innovation_11d960b7-en

16 Be Belmont, J.W., Hardenbol, P., Willis, T.D., Yu, F., Yang, H., Ch'Ang, L.Y., Huang, W., Liu, B., Shen, Y., Tam, P.K.H. and Tsui, L.C., 2003. The international HapMap project. *Nature*, 426(6968), pp.789–796; Campbell, P.J., Getz, G., Korbel, J.O., Stuart, J.M., Jennings, J.L. and Stein, L.D., Pan-cancer analysis of whole genomes. Nature [Internet]. 2020; 578 (7793): 82–93; Maxson Jones, K., Ankeny, R. and Cook-Deegan, R., 2018. The Bermuda Triangle: the pragmatics, policies, and principles for data sharing in the history of the human genome. *Journal of the History of Biology*, 51(4), pp. 1–113.

17 Garden, H., Hawkins, N. and Winickoff, D., 2021. Building and sustaining collaborative platforms in genomics and biobanks for health innovation. *OECD Science, Technology and Industry Policy Papers*, No. 102, OECD Publishing, Paris. https://www.oecd-ilibrary.org/science-and-technology/building-and-sustaining-collaborative-platforms-in-genomics-and-biobanks-for-health-innovation_11d960b7-en

18 Mitchell, M., 2019. *Artificial Intelligence: A Guide for Thinking Humans*. Penguin, London, UK.

19 Dou, Q., So, T.Y., Jiang, M., Liu, Q., Vardhanabhuti, V., Kaissis, G., Li, Z., Si, W., Lee, H.H., Yu, K. and Feng, Z., 2021. Federated deep learning for detecting COVID-19 lung abnormalities in CT: a privacy-preserving multinational validation study. *NPJ Digital Medicine*, 4(1), p. 60.

20 ImageNet. http://www.image-net.org/. Accessed November 21, 2018.

21 Brodley, C.E. and Friedl, M.A., 1999. Identifying mislabeled training data. *Journal of Artificial Intelligence Research*, 11, pp. 131–167; Boutell, M.R., Luo, J., Shen, X. and Brown, C.M., 2004. Learning multi-label scene classification. *Pattern Recognition*, 37(9), pp. 1757–1771; Roy, S., Menapace, W., Oei, S., Luijten, B., Fini, E., Saltori, C., Huijben, I., Chennakeshava, N., Mento, F., Sentelli, A. and Peschiera, E., 2020. Deep learning for classification and localization of COVID-19 markers in point-of-care lung ultrasound. *IEEE Transactions on Medical Imaging*, 39(8), pp. 2676–2687.

22 Kahneman, Sibony, O. and Sunstein, C.R. 2021. *Noise: A Flaw in Human Judgement*. New York: Little, Brown Spark.

23 Wang, X., Peng, Y., Lu, L., Lu, Z., Bagheri, M. and Summers, R.M., 2017. Chestx-ray8: Hospital-scale chest X-ray database and benchmarks on weakly-supervised classification and localization of common thorax diseases. In *Proceedings of the IEEE Conference on Computer Vision and Pattern Recognition* (pp. 2097–2106), IEEE, Hawaii, USA.

24 Darzidehkalani, E., Ghasemi-Rad, M. and van Ooijen, P.M.A., 2022. Federated learning in medical imaging: Part I: toward multicentral health care ecosystems. *Journal of the American College of Radiology*, 19(8), pp. 969–974.

25 https://c3.ai/glossary/machine-learning/ground-truth/; also see Lebovitz, S., Levina, N. and Lifshitz-Assaf, H., 2021. Is AI ground truth really 'true'? The dangers of training and evaluating AI tools based on experts' know-what. *MIS Quarterly*, 45(3), pp. 1501–1526; Xu, J., Yang, P., Xue, S., Sharma, B., Sanchez-Martin, M., Wang, F., Beaty, K.A., Dehan, E. and Parikh, B., 2019. Translating cancer genomics into precision medicine with artificial intelligence: applications, challenges and future perspectives. *Human Genetics*, 138(2), pp. 109–124.

26 https://www.cancer.org/cancer/breast-cancer/about/how-common-is-breast-cancer.html; https://www.nhs.uk/conditions/breast-cancer/

27 https://research.ibm.com/blog/what-are-foundation-models

28 Diao, E., Ding, J. and Tarokh, V., 2020. HeteroFL: computation and communication efficient federated learning for heterogeneous clients. *arXiv preprint arXiv:2010.01264*.

29 Kairouz, P., McMahan, H.B., Avent, B., Bellet, A., Bennis, M., Bhagoji, A.N., Bonawitz, K., Charles, Z., Cormode, G., Cummings, R. and D'Oliveira, R.G., 2021. Advances and open problems in federated learning. *Foundations and Trends® in Machine Learning*, 14(1–2), pp. 1–210.

30 Garden, H., Hawkins, N. and Winickoff, D. 2021. Building and sustaining collaborative platforms in genomics and biobanks for health innovation, *OECD Science, Technology and Industry Policy Papers*, No. 102, OECD Publishing, Paris. https://www.oecd-ilibrary.org/science-and-technology/building-and-sustaining-collaborative-platforms-in-genomics-and-biobanks-for-health-innovation_11d960b7-en

31 Budd, J., Miller, B.S., Manning, E.M., Lampos, V., Zhuang, M., Edelstein, M., Rees, G., Emery, V.C., Stevens, M.M., Keegan, N. and Short, M.J., 2020. Digital technologies in the public-health response to COVID-19. *Nature Medicine*, 26(8), pp. 1183–1192; Moorthy, V., Restrepo, A.M.H., Preziosi, M.P. and Swaminathan, S., 2020. Data sharing for novel coronavirus (COVID-19). *Bulletin of the World Health Organization*, 98(3), p. 150.

32 Dayan, I., Roth, H.R., Zhong, A., Harouni, A., Gentili, A., Abidin, A.Z., Liu, A., Costa, A.B., Wood, B.J., Tsai, C.S. and Wang, C.H., 2021. Federated learning for predicting clinical outcomes in patients with COVID-19. *Nature Medicine*, 27(10), pp. 1735–1743.

33 Buch, V., Zhong, A., Li, X., Rockenbach, M.A.B.C., Wu, D., Ren, H., Guan, J., Liteplo, A., Dutta, S., Dayan, I. and Li, Q., 2021. Development and validation of a deep learning model for prediction of severe outcomes in suspected COVID-19 infection. *arXiv preprint arXiv:2103.11269*. https://europepmc.org/article/ppr/ppr342992

34 Dayan, I., Roth, H.R., Zhong, A., Harouni, A., Gentili, A., Abidin, A.Z., Liu, A., Costa, A.B., Wood, B.J., Tsai, C.S. and Wang, C.H., 2021. Federated learning for predicting clinical outcomes in patients with COVID-19. *Nature Medicine*, 27(10), pp. 1735–1743. p.1738.

35 Ibid. p. 1735.

36 https://www.lifebit.ai/

37 Barja, P.P., Chatzou, M., Sosic, M., Sosic, M., Silva, D.N.P., Goncalves, B.F.R., De Jesus, T.F.S., Kruglova, O. and Dobrev, D., Lifebit Biotech Ltd, 2020. *Federated Computational Analysis over Distributed Data*. U.S. Patent 10,769,167.

38 UK Health Data Research Alliance & NHSX. (2021) *Building Trusted Research Environments –Principles and Best Practices; Towards TRE ecosystems*. https://ukhealthdata.org/projects/aligning-approach-to-trusted-research-environments/

39 https://www.hdruk.ac.uk/

40 https://www.opensafely.org/

41 https://www.genomicsengland.co.uk/research/research-environment

42 https://www.ohdsi.org/data-standardization/

43 https://www.ibm.com/topics/elt

44 https://www.okta.com/uk/

45 https://auth0.com/

46 Rehm, H.L., Page, A.J., Smith, L., Adams, J.B., Alterovitz, G., Babb, L.J., Barkley, M.P., Baudis, M., Beauvais, M.J., Beck, T. and Beckmann, J.S., 2021. GA4GH: International policies and standards for data sharing across genomic research and healthcare. *Cell Genomics*, 1(2), p. 100029

47 https://www.lifebit.ai/white-papers/lifebit-approach-to-data-governance-security

48 https://re-docs.genomicsengland.co.uk/airlock/

49 https://www.lifebit.ai/white-papers/top-10-best-practices-building-trusted-research-environment

50 https://dareuk.org.uk/about/

51 https://dareuk.org.uk/sprint-exemplar-project-multi-party-trusted-research-environment-federation/

52 Cell Genomics. (2021). *GA4GH: International Policies and Standards for Data Sharing across Genomic Research and Healthcare*. Retrieved from https://www.cell.com/cell-genomics/fulltext/S2666-979X(21)00036-7

53 Wilkinson, M.D., Dumontier, M., Aalbersberg, I.J., Appleton, G., Axton, M., Baak, A., Blomberg, N., Boiten, J.W., da Silva Santos, L.B., Bourne, P.E. and Bouwman, J., 2016. The FAIR guiding principles for scientific data management and stewardship. *Scientific Data*, 3(1), pp. 1–9.

54 Wu, B., Zhao, S., Sun, G., Zhang, X., Su, Z., Zeng, C. and Liu, Z., 2019. P3sgd: patient privacy preserving SGD for regularizing deep CNNS in pathological image classification. In *Proceedings of the IEEE/CVF Conference on Computer Vision and Pattern Recognition* (pp. 2099–2108), IEEE, California, USA.

55 Zhao, Z., Luo, M. and Ding, W., 2022. Deep leakage from model in federated learning. *arXiv preprint arXiv:2206.04887.* https://arxiv.org/pdf/2206.04887.pdf

56 Melis, L., Song, C., De Cristofaro, E. and Shmatikov, V., 2018. Inference attacks against collaborative learning. *arXiv preprint arXiv:1805.04049, 13.* https://arxiv.org/pdf/1805.04049.pdf

57 Bagdasaryan, E., Veit, A., Hua, Y., Estrin, D. and Shmatikov, V., 2020, June. How to backdoor federated learning. In *International Conference on Artificial Intelligence and Statistics* (pp. 2938–2948). PMLR. https://proceedings.mlr.press/v108/ Held Online.

58 Mishra, A.K., Tripathy, A.K., Puthal, D. and Yang, L.T., 2018. Analytical model for sybil attack phases in internet of things. *IEEE Internet of Things Journal, 6(1),* pp. 379–387.

59 Wang, Z., Song, M., Zhang, Z., Song, Y., Wang, Q. and Qi, H., 2019, April. Beyond inferring class representatives: user-level privacy leakage from federated learning. In *IEEE INFOCOM 2019-IEEE Conference on Computer Communications* (pp. 2512–2520). IEEE, Paris, France.

60 Aouedi, O., Sacco, A., Piamrat, K. and Marchetto, G., 2022. Handling privacy-sensitive medical data with federated learning: challenges and future directions. *IEEE Journal of Biomedical and Health Informatics, 27(2),* pp. 790–803.

61 Dayan, I., Roth, H.R., Zhong, A., Harouni, A., Gentili, A., Abidin, A.Z., Liu, A., Costa, A.B., Wood, B.J., Tsai, C.S. and Wang, C.H., 2021. Federated learning for predicting clinical outcomes in patients with COVID-19. *Nature Medicine, 27(10),* pp. 1735–1743.

62 Zeggini, E., Gloyn, A.L., Barton, A.C. and Wain, L.V., 2019. Translational genomics and precision medicine: moving from the lab to the clinic. *Science, 365(6460),* pp. 1409–1413.

63 Ginsburg, G.S. and Phillips, K.A., 2018. Precision medicine: from science to value. *Health Affairs, 37(5),* pp. 694–701.

64 Ostrom, E., 1990. *Governing the Commons: The Evolution of institutions for Collective Action.* Cambridge University Press., Cambridge UK.

65 Fenech, M., Strukelj, N. and Buston, O., 2018. Ethical, social, and political challenges of artificial intelligence in health. London: Wellcome Trust Future Advocacy, 12. https://wellcome.org/sites/default/files/ai-in-health-ethical-social-political-challenges.pdf

66 Kraft, S.A., Cho, M.K., Gillespie, K., Halley, M., Varsava, N., Ormond, K.E., Luft, H.S., Wilfond, B.S. and Lee, S.S.J., 2018. Beyond consent: building trusting relationships with diverse populations in precision medicine research. *The American Journal of Bioethics, 18(4),* pp. 3–20.

67 Fenech, M., Strukelj, N. and Buston, O., 2018. Ethical, social, and political challenges of artificial intelligence in health. London: Wellcome Trust Future Advocacy, 12. https://wellcome.org/sites/default/files/ai-in-health-ethical-social-political-challenges.pdf

68 Dheensa, S., Lucassen, A. and Fenwick, A., 2019. Fostering trust in healthcare: participants' experiences, views, and concerns about the 100,000 genomes project. *European Journal of Medical Genetics, 62(5),* pp. 335–341.

69 Milne, R., Morley, K.I., Howard, H., Niemiec, E., Nicol, D., Critchley, C., Prainsack, B., Vears, D., Smith, J., Steed, C. and Bevan, P., 2019. Trust in genomic data sharing among members of the general public in the UK, USA, Canada and Australia. *Human Genetics, 138,* pp. 1237–1246.; IPSOS MORI for Wellcome Trust, I. (2016), *The One-Way Mirror: Public Attitudes to Commercial Access to Health Data,* Ipsos MORI Social Research Institute https://www.ipsos.com/sites/default/files/publication/5200-03/sri-wellcome-trust-commercial-access-to-health-data.pdf, London, UK.

70 World Economic Forum (WEF) (2020), *Genomic Data Policy Framework and Ethical Tensions,* http://www.weforum.org

71 Dreyfuss, R.C., Nielsen, J. and Nicol, D., 2018. Patenting nature—a comparative perspective. *Journal of Law and the Biosciences, 5(3),* pp. 550–589.

72 Aboy, M., Crespo, C., Liddell, K., Minssen, T. and Liddicoat, J., 2019. Mayo's impact on patent applications related to biotechnology, diagnostics and personalized medicine. *Nature Biotechnology, 37(5),* pp. 513–518.

73 Liddell, K., Liddicoat, J. and Jordan, M., 2019. IP policies for large bioresources: the fiction, fantasy, and future of openness. In Minssen, T., Herrmann, J.R. and Schovsbo, J. (eds.) *Global Genes, Local Concerns* (pp. 242–263). Edward Elgar Publishing, London, UK.

74 Van Overwalle, G. ed., 2009. *Gene Patents and Collaborative Licensing Models: Patent Pools, Clearinghouses, Open Source Models and Liability Regimes.* Cambridge University Press, Cambridge, UK; Graff, G.D. and Sherkow, J.S., 2020. Models of technology transfer for genome-editing technologies. *Annual Review of Genomics and Human Genetics*, 21, pp. 509–534.

75 https://www.who.int/initiatives/covid-19-technology-access-pool

76 Hawkins, N., 2020. Patents and non-invasive prenatal testing: is there cause for concern?. *Science and Public Policy*, 47(5), pp. 655–667.

Part 3

Generative Transformation, The Race to Tech Arms and Regulation

Part 3 concludes the book by discussing the recent coming of age of generative AI technologies, such as OpenAI's Chat GPT-4 and Microsoft's Bing AI and 365 Copilot.

Chapter 7 provides an analysis of this very turbulent landscape and discusses ways by which organizations can navigate digital transformation by using generative AI technologies. The chapter provides a discussion of both the possibilities and challenges of generative AI in healthcare, before diving deep into the race to tech arms between big tech companies, open-source developers and healthcare organizations. The chapter concludes by examining recent regulation on AI technologies and makes a set of proposals for technology policy to govern generative AI in healthcare.

DOI: 10.4324/9781032619569-9

7   Generative Transformation and Regulatory Challenges

When OpenAI's GPT-3 was publicly released in November 2022, it took the world by storm. The introduction of this technology signaled a significant milestone, the coming of age of generative AI, with the potential to transform a wide range of sectors, including healthcare. Currently, a number of companies including Microsoft,[1] Google,[2] Tencent and Baidu,[3] as well as open-source developers on GitHub.[4] are developing generative AI technologies for text, audio, video and image generation, software programming and other developer tools, as well as more specialized services for existing digital platforms.

Generative AI can understand and process text-based language queries. This forms a ground-breaking interface to interacting with advanced technologies, moving beyond the confines of specialized facilities, data analytics software packages and expert computer engineers. Generative AI is conversational, meaning that anyone, even lay users, can ask simple questions, receive comprehensive answers and make informed decisions about a number of different tasks. In healthcare, generative AI can interface with other technologies including electronic patient records, diagnostic devices such as MRI and CT scanners, laboratory systems and many more, leveraging heterogeneous datasets and augmenting healthcare professionals to make more informed decisions across the healthcare delivery cycle.

Generative AI has created a lot of hype as to the potential to positively transform healthcare services. What makes this technology unique and orders of magnitude more transformative than any other technology that has come before it is the fact that it can learn from billions of data points and interact with millions of users simultaneously. It can read all the electronic care records, all the published research, all doctor notes, all diagnostic exams and so on and can filter through all that data to produce original outcomes of relevance to multiple users.

At the same time, exactly because of the scale and speed generative AI can perform it has raised concerns of the possible systemic risks it carries especially if the technology is controlled by actors with malicious intentions. In addition, exactly because generative AI technologies such as Open AI's ChatGPT rely on a predictive model, they are constantly trying to be accurate, but not necessarily reliable and valid.[5] There are also significant challenges related to the ownership and control of the global models driving individual generative AI technologies like OpenAI's GPT-4, but also control over the data being generated by these technologies. Big tech companies like Google, Amazon, Microsoft, Tencent and Baidu have the financial resources and technical power to control not only the generative AI technologies themselves but also the data being generated through them.[6] These big tech companies also own many cloud-adjacent technology markets

DOI: 10.4324/9781032619569-10

such as edge, 5G and the Internet of Medical Things, which offer the tools with which to process and analyze data, enabling decision-making across administrative, operational and clinical tasks.

This control raises important questions about who benefits from this new wave of generative AI technologies and who is at risk of being left behind. On the one hand, big tech companies are in competition with one another, seeking to control the technologies that can revolutionize healthcare services in the future. On the other hand, other ecosystem actors such as hospitals, private and public payers of healthcare services, employers and even national governments are in a Red Queen race, trying to catch up to the big tech companies. They can either join the big tech companies or be consumed by them. These organizations are becoming increasingly reliant on big tech companies both in relation to technological choices, but also in relation to how data produced internally becomes analyzed and accessed by third parties. This race to tech arms will have consequences for the future of the global healthcare sector, including the way patients access and use healthcare services.

Regulatory authorities across regions have a huge task to ensure a healthy competition without hurting innovation and while protecting patients from harm that may arise due to unsafe technological solutions. This chapter provides an analysis of this very turbulent landscape and discusses ways by which organizations can navigate digital transformation. The chapter examines recent regulation on AI technologies, discusses the challenges involved and makes a set of proposals for technology policy to govern generative AI in healthcare.

7.1   Generative AI and the Disruption of Traditional Boundaries

7.1.1   *The Potential of Generative AI in Healthcare*

Generative AI is a powerful technology that has gained significant attention in recent years. It has been a focused area of AI research since 2014,[7] while large language models date back to 1980s when they were used as components for automatic speech recognition, machine translation, document classification and many more.[8] However, generative AI technologies only took off in 2022 when the technology was put into the hands of consumers with the release of text-to-image models like DALL-E 2 and Stable Diffusion, text-to-video systems like Make-A-Video, and chatbots like GPT-4, among many more.[9] These technologies are scaling fast in terms of their computing power and neural network architectures, and researchers are exploring new ways to train them with larger and more diverse datasets. This trend is leading to remarkable advancements in generative AI, especially in healthcare.

One of the key advantages of generative AI is that it can understand and interpret human language through natural language processing (NLP). NLP can be used to analyze vast amounts of various types of medical data, while allowing users to ask questions in a conversational style, as if having a personal machine agent.[10] This agent will be able to help with scheduling, communications and commercial transactions, but also analytical and presentation tasks, and it will work across all devices and applications. For example, Microsoft has introduced Copilot,[11] a generative AI technology that can assist users of Office 365 applications in different tasks. Administrative personnel and nursing staff will be augmented with tasks such as filing insurance claims, dealing with paperwork, and drafting notes from a doctor's visit. All of this will help improve productivity and address the global shortage of healthcare professionals.[12]

In addition, researchers are exploring the use of generative AI in a number of applications that can help improve the quality of healthcare services across the healthcare delivery cycle. For example, generative AI can be trained to generate high-quality images of prostate cancer from 2D MRI images.[13] These synthetic images can help overcome the challenge of limited availability of medical images, especially in rare diseases or specific imaging modalities.

Generative AI can also help to accelerate the drug discovery process by analyzing large datasets and identifying potential new drug candidates. AI-powered simulations can predict the efficacy of a drug, reducing the time and costs associated with clinical trials. For example, traditional methods for antibody discovery offer little control over the outputs with the consequence that proposed antibodies are often suboptimal generating huge costs for pharmaceutical companies. Using generative AI technologies a team of researchers managed to create antibodies with a single round of model generation without further optimizations.[14] These AI-generated antibodies are more robust than antibodies generated through traditional methods accelerating the process of drug discovery.

These generative AI technologies can quickly and easily integrate with existing AI systems exactly because of their conversational interface. For example, generative AI technologies can integrate with AI systems to develop personalized treatment plans for individual patients based on their unique genetic and medical history. By analyzing large datasets, AI can identify the most effective treatments for each patient, reducing the risk of adverse reactions and improving patient outcomes. Biotech companies like BenevolentAI are partnering with pharmaceutical companies to discover novel treatments based on a patient's genetic biomarkers.[15] Further, generative AI technologies can integrate with predictive analytics software from companies like Mendelian[16] and Cogito[17] to identify patients at risk of developing certain conditions, enabling healthcare providers to intervene early and prevent the onset of disease. Such AI solutions can also be used to monitor patients with chronic conditions, such as diabetes and heart disease, to improve disease management and reduce the risk of complications. Finally, generative AI can integrate with existing AI chatbots to give patients the ability to do basic triage, get advice about how to deal with health problems and decide whether they need to seek treatment. For example, there are already numerous AI chatbots that help patients triage for basic symptoms,[18] AI tools that can detect dermatological cancer[19] and AI technologies that can read ultrasounds and deliver recommendations on mobile phones.[20]

These are just a few examples of the potential applications of generative AI technologies in healthcare. By improving diagnosis, treatment and prevention, these technologies have the potential to improve patient outcomes, reduce healthcare costs and digitally transform the healthcare delivery cycle.

7.1.2 The Challenges of Generative AI in Healthcare

Despite the remarkable progress made in generative AI, there are still significant challenges that need to be addressed. One such challenge is the lack of transparency in how these technologies work. As these technologies scale and become more complex, it becomes increasingly difficult to understand how they produce different outcomes. This issue is particularly concerning in the healthcare sector, where the stakes are high and the consequences of errors can be life-threatening. As such, it is essential to understand how these models arrive at their decisions to ensure that they are safe and effective.

Generative AI technologies are often based on complex algorithms and neural network architectures that are difficult for humans to understand and that is why they are often referred to as "black boxes".[21] In many cases, even the developers of these systems may not fully understand how they work or why they produce certain outputs. This lack of transparency can make it difficult to verify the accuracy and trustworthiness of these technologies. For example, a study[22] by Mount Sinai Hospital in New York used an AI neural network with 700,000 electronic patient records. Without any expert instruction, the neural network had discovered patterns hidden in the data that seemed to indicate when people were on the way to a wide range of ailments, including cancer of the liver. At the same time, the neural network predicted the onset of psychiatric disorders like schizophrenia, which has been notoriously difficult for doctors to predict. The neural network offered no explanation as to how it was able to come to this outcome something which was challenged by doctors.[23] Another study[24] used an AI neural network to predict which hospitalized patients with pneumonia were at high risk of serious complications. The neural network wrongly predicted that asthmatics do better with pneumonia, potentially instructing doctors to send the patients with asthma home. What this example shows is that there is a difference between receiving a statistical result without any explanations as to how the neural network reached this result, and what we now see becoming a trend in AI which is the ability to build causality in the steps taken to reach that result.[25] Understanding why and how a given outcome was reached is paramount in gaining the trust of the end user – the doctors, but also the patients.

One of the biggest concerns about the lack of transparency in generative AI in healthcare is the potential for bias embedded in large datasets.[26] These technologies depend on large datasets collected from the web such as the Colossal Clean Crawled Corpus, the Pile, Wikipedia and Reddit among others. One would think that these large datasets are representative of diverse communities, perspectives and beliefs. However, research has already shown that Internet access is not evenly distributed, resulting in Internet data over-representing younger users and those from developed countries.[27] Indeed, certain views (e.g., white supremacist, misogynistic, ageist, etc.) are overrepresented in these data. As others have noted, "in accepting large amounts of web text as 'representative' of 'all' of humanity we risk perpetuating dominant viewpoints, increasing power imbalances, and further reifying inequality".[28] For example, one study found that an AI system used to predict which patients would benefit from extra care in the US healthcare system was less accurate for Black patients than for white patients.[29] This type of bias can lead to significant disparities in healthcare outcomes and perpetuate existing inequalities.

Another concern is the potential for errors in generative AI to go undetected, leading to incorrect diagnoses or treatment recommendations. For example, a recent study found that AI systems used to predict the severity of COVID-19 based on chest X-rays were found to be unreliable, with significant errors in some cases.[30] If such errors are not detected, they could lead to patients receiving incorrect treatment or being overlooked for necessary care. These errors are once again related to data. As discussed in Chapter 6, lack of data on different modalities, different types of patients and normal vs rare cases can all lead to either overfitting (establishing "ground truth" around cases that are most prevalent in the dataset) or underfitting (failing to establish "ground truth" altogether because of lack of appropriate data). Data cleaning, annotation and validation are all processes that can suffer from bad quality data leading to errors.

The lack of transparency in generative AI in healthcare also raises important ethical questions. For example, doctors can prompt generative AI technology to help them interpret novel medical cases. However, if doctors follow the technology's recommendation, who should be held responsible if something goes wrong?[31] Should it be the developers of the AI system, the healthcare providers who used it, or the patients who agreed to use the model's recommendations? These types of questions highlight the need for transparency and accountability in the development and use of AI systems in healthcare[32] and is a topic discussed extensively in section 7.4.

In addition, training these large generative AI technologies with a deep neural network architecture has high development costs, both in terms of money spent and estimated CO_2 emissions.[33] For example, the average person is responsible for an estimated 5t CO_2 per year, while some generative AI models are estimated to emit 284t of CO_2. Further, most of this generative AI technology is built to serve the needs of those who have the financial resources to purchase such devices as a Google Home, an Amazon Alexa or an Apple device and to access high speed broadband Internet through which to access technologies such as GPT-4. Such "environmental racism" impacts the less privileged, marginalized communities around the world.[34]

Finally, one of the biggest challenges that is not quite visible yet, though it will be the most disruptive on the healthcare workforce, is the fact that generative AI technologies are improving their performance by orders of magnitude faster than humans alone and even by humans with other technologies. For example, researchers from Microsoft and Open AI have carried out a comprehensive evaluation of the performance of GPT-4 on the United States Medical Licensing Examination (USMLE).[35] The results are based on sample exams and self-assessment materials officially published by the National Board of Medical Examiners (NBME). The findings show that GPT-4 significantly outperforms earlier models, achieving an average score of 86.65% and 86.7% on the self-assessment and sample exam of the USMLE tests, respectively, compared to 53.61% and 58.78% for GPT-3.5, that was released 6 months earlier. GPT-4 has exhibited a similarly impressive performance on several other tests including AP Chemistry, AP Biology, SAT Math and many more.[36]

A recent study examined the impact of GPT-4 and other generative AI technologies on the labor market and found that "up to 49% of workers could have half or more of their tasks exposed" to these technologies.[37] What this means is that these "exposed tasks" could be either augmented or automated[38] by generative AI technologies. Human experts working with these technologies will have their tasks augmented, that is, optimized, improved or better performed. Others, however, will have their tasks automated, meaning that their jobs may be displaced. Other research has argued that, historically, the introduction of new, general-purpose technologies creates new types of task and new types of jobs and that we should be careful not to hit the panic button that AI will steal our jobs.[39] Yet, generative AI technologies have the capability to improve their performance exponentially, and this improvement is accentuated with their integration with complementary technologies. What this means is that the cost of human cognition and of creative work increasingly drops to zero. If these technologies can do the work of many – not just a single human – at a speed and scale that is unimaginable for humans and at a near zero cost of employment[40] would employers choose humans over machines?

Many of the aforementioned challenges are not easy to address, at least not immediately, because the impact of the disruption has not been felt yet by those most concerned. Certainly, many experts have started raising concerns already and calling for structural and processual changes that would help regulate generative AI as discussed in section 7.3. Not everyone agrees, however, especially as the race to own and control these generative

AI technologies intensifies. While big tech companies want to have the competitive advantage over how these technologies are developed and deployed, other ecosystem actors such as hospitals, private and public payers of healthcare services, employers and even national governments are in a Red Queen race, trying to forge partnerships that would help them build defensive moats over valuable resources. This race to tech arms will significantly impact the way patients access and use healthcare services.

7.2   The Race to Tech Arms in Healthcare

At the forefront of this race are the big tech companies such as Google, Amazon, Microsoft, Tencent and Alibaba, who are investing heavily in developing and acquiring AI technologies for healthcare. These companies have significant financial resources, technical expertise and massive amounts of data at their disposal, giving them a competitive advantage over other ecosystem actors. Indeed, these big tech companies have significant influence over the development of generative AI through their investments in research and development. One recent study has found that big tech AI systems are 29 times bigger, on average, than academic ones, highlighting the vast difference in computing power available to the two groups.[41] The same study found that big tech companies have an ability to hire talent and leverage greater computing power because of differences in spending. Also, research papers with one or more co-authors from big tech have grown from 22% in 2000 to 38% in 2020.

The dominance of big tech in new generative AI in healthcare is evident in recent business developments. For example, Google recently announced a new AI-powered health division, Google Health, which aims to develop and deploy AI technologies for a range of healthcare applications. Google Health has already launched a range of AI-powered tools, such as Google's DeepMind Health[42] division that has been working on developing AI systems to help detect and diagnose conditions such as breast cancer and diabetic retinopathy. The company has access to a large dataset of mammograms and retinal scans, which it can use to train and improve its AI systems. In addition, DeepMind's AlphaFold[43] technology has cataloged 200 million protein structures accelerating research in chronic disease detection, drug discovery and personalized medicine.

Others like Amazon and Microsoft are also investing heavily in healthcare AI technologies, with their cloud computing platforms. Amazon Web Services for Health is offering a range of AI-powered tools and services for healthcare providers. Amazon has also acquired PillPack, an online pharmacy, and has announced plans to launch a primary care service for its employees. Microsoft is also heavily involved in healthcare AI, with its Healthcare NExT initiative focusing on developing AI technologies for precision medicine, disease prevention and personalized care. Microsoft has also partnered with hospitals and healthcare providers to develop AI-powered solutions for a range of healthcare applications. Most notably, Microsoft has recently announced that they are "expanding their long-standing strategic collaboration to develop and integrate generative AI into healthcare by combining the scale and power of Azure OpenAI Service with Epic's industry-leading electronic health record (EHR) software".[44] In the same announcement, Epic's senior vice president of research and development said that, "Our exploration of OpenAI's GPT-4 has shown the potential to increase the power and accessibility of self-service reporting through SlicerDicer, making it easier for healthcare organizations to identify operational improvements, including ways to reduce costs and to find answers to questions locally and in a broader context".

Having big tech companies control generative AI technologies and the data they generate can help further refine these technologies at a faster pace than smaller competitors, leading to faster advancements and greater innovation. At the same time, the control over generative AI by big tech companies raises concerns of fair competition across all stakeholders, including smaller organizations, patients and society as a whole. The commercial interests of big tech companies can lead to an increased lack of transparency in the development and use of generative AI, as discussed in the previous section. Furthermore, the data generated by generative AI technologies is incredibly valuable, and the companies that control this data have significant power and influence. For example, Amazon's control over customer data through its Amazon Prime, Amazon Web Services, Amazon Marketplace and Alexa voice assistant has given the company a significant advantage in potentially disrupting the virtual health market.[45]

Although healthcare organizations may be hesitant to share their data, they may find themselves unable to resist the new wave of transformation by generative AI technologies, especially as many of them depend on such strategic partners as Epic for their electronic health records. Big tech companies have faced criticism in the past for their handling of user data, and the use of healthcare data is particularly sensitive.[46] This lack of transparency can have significant implications for the fair and ethical use of generative AI, especially as decisions produced by these technologies across the healthcare delivery cycle remain black-boxed.

Fortunately, it is not just big tech companies that are competing in this race. Open-source developers are increasingly experimenting with copies of generative AI technologies, tinkering them and producing impressive results. For example, OpenAI's DALL-E, a generative AI technology used to create synthetic images, was released in January 2021 but was overpowered by Stable Diffusion, the open source version released a year and a half later in August 2022. A leaked memo by a senior software engineer at Google admits that "While our models still hold a slight edge in terms of quality, the gap is closing astonishingly quickly. Open-source models are faster, more customizable, more private, and pound-for-pound more capable. They are doing things with $100 and 13B params that we struggle with at $10M and 540B. And they are doing so in weeks, not months".[47] The memo notes that while Google and other big tech have made significant investments in generative AI research and development, they may not have a "moat" or a sustainable competitive advantage in this area, as open-source communities are also developing similar technologies. In fact, the memo suggests that open-source developers may be able to address the problem of scale in developing these technologies more effectively than Google, as they can leverage the collective efforts of a global community of developers. The question and answer dataset used to create the open-source clone technology, Dolly 2.0, was entirely created by thousands of volunteers. Google and OpenAI relied partially on question and answers, scraped from sites like Reddit, something that, as discussed earlier, creates issues of data quality. The open-source question and answer dataset is claimed to be of a higher quality because the humans who contributed to creating it were professionals, and the answers they provided were longer and more substantial than what is found in a typical question and answer dataset scraped from a public forum. The memo notes that new machine learning techniques such as LoRA (Low-Rank Adaptation of Large Language Models) enable optimizations in a matter of days with exceedingly low cost, especially when compared with the exceedingly more expensive technologies created by Google and OpenAI.

Certainly, the negative implications of the democratization of generative AI technology, particularly with regards to the ability to generate high-quality synthetic text at scale, involve risks of fake news and misinformation, but also cyberattacks on broader social and political institutions. As extensively discussed in Chapters 4–6, the biggest challenge of open-source platform ecosystems is that, the ecosystem orchestrator (usually a community or consortium of organizations) has a limited ability to enforce common governance rules, which may end up in a "tragedy of the commons".[48] Individuals and communities may act opportunistically, some with malicious intentions, others purely seeking to serve their self-interests, and yet others simply ignoring commonly agreed rules of participation that eventually hurt the ecosystem. This is why "benevolent dictators" are needed to ensure successful coordination between ecosystem actors.[49] In an open-source project, a key individual, acting as the leading figure, addressing disputes and setting strategic objectives may be sufficient, as the case of Linus Torvalds and the Linux Kernel project has shown, but also many others.[50] However, for bigger, more heterogeneous ecosystems, with multiple digital transformation projects running at the same time, an institutional actor is needed to act as an ecosystem orchestrator to help coordinate the governance of co-innovation and co-adoption risks.

Hospitals, private and public payers of healthcare services, employers and national governments are all relevant actors that can join forces and act as ecosystem orchestrators. They can work with open-source developers to create strong ecosystems that can compete with the big tech companies. Evidently, organizations with access to large and diverse datasets will have a competitive advantage to developing and training generative AI technologies that can augment processes across the healthcare delivery cycle. In addition, organizations with strong technical capabilities in machine learning, natural language processing and data analytics as applied in specific healthcare services will be better positioned to develop and implement generative AI tools. More importantly, organizations that own or can protect their generative AI technology through patents, copyrights or other means will also have a competitive advantage in the market and will be attractive to other ecosystem actors in the development of partnerships. Finally, organizations with deep pockets and access to financial resources will be better positioned to make investments in research and development, infrastructure and talent acquisition.

Effectively, this race to tech arms in generative AI constitutes a new cycle of digital transformation across the healthcare delivery cycle. As discussed in Chapter 3, those organizations with a higher level of digital maturity will be better positioned to make the necessary changes to swiftly transform to new AI-enabled services. They will be in a position to either orchestrate new platform ecosystems or become strategic partners in other ecosystems. Organizations with low digital maturity, high technical debt and limited resources will struggle to catch up with this new wave of digital transformation and may have little bargaining power as to how resources are allocated, deployed and used.

This is also true for individual patients. Those empowered to take hold of their own health and well-being through the use of personal devices and sensors and who can afford to do so will benefit the most. As more personal technologies diffuse across different population segments and as more digital data is generated by individuals, there are increased opportunities for developing new generative AI technologies for personalized medicine. However, some patients, those who cannot even get access to conventional healthcare services, let alone services augmented by generative AI, will benefit the least from this race. Unfortunately, as evident from previous industrial revolutions, technological transformations tend to aggravate inequalities among populations.

In summary, the race to tech arms in generative AI is driven by the potential for significant financial and strategic benefits, as well as the fear of being left behind for the losers. Big tech companies such as Google, Amazon and Microsoft are leading the charge, but other ecosystem actors are also investing heavily in AI technologies to catch up. The winners of this race will have significant influence over the future of healthcare, with the potential to revolutionize the industry and improve patient outcomes. Now, more than ever, the need for *generative* not static regulation is needed if we want to avoid mistakes of the past, while helping to address known inequalities, user harm, as well as harm to fair competition. While technology-neutral laws, such as non-discrimination law, and also data protection law, continue to apply to these new generative AI technologies, as they do apply in other technologies, there seems to be a trend toward technology-specific rules enforced as a blanket regulation. The next section discusses the challenges with current regulation.

7.3 Challenges of Regulating Generative AI in Healthcare

On March 22, 2023, a number of prominent AI experts, tech entrepreneurs and scientists called on *"all AI labs to immediately pause for at least 6 months the training of AI systems more powerful than GPT-4"* in an open letter.[51] The letter was published by the non-profit Future of Life Institute[52] which was founded to "reduce global catastrophic and existential risk from powerful technologies" with founders coming from MIT and DeepMind. The open letter against generative AI says that *"With more data and compute, the capabilities of AI systems are scaling rapidly. The largest models are increasingly capable of surpassing human performance across many domains. No single company can forecast what this means for our societies."* The letter points out that superintelligence is far from the only harm to be concerned about when it comes to generative AI, the potential for impersonation and disinformation are others.[53] However, it does emphasize that the stated goal of many commercial labs is to develop AGI (artificial general intelligence) and adds that some researchers believe that we are close to AGI, with accompanying concerns for AGI safety and ethics.

Other prominent AI scientists argued against a proposed pause on the development of generative AI technologies arguing that *"There are probably several motivations from the various signatories of that letter"*,[54] including commercial interests, as discussed in the previous sections. Some of these motivations *"are, perhaps on one extreme, worried about AGI being turned on and then eliminating humanity on short notice. I think few people really believe in this kind of scenario, or believe it's a definite threat that cannot be stopped"*, said Yann LeCun, Silver Professor of the Courant Institute of Mathematical Sciences at New York University and Vice President, Chief AI Scientist at Meta. *"Then there are people who are more reasonable, who think that there is real potential harm and danger that needs to be dealt with — and I agree with them"*, he continued. Andrew Ng, formerly associate professor and Director of the Stanford AI Lab and cofounder of both Coursera and Deeplearning.ai, who also participated in the live discussion added that regulation is necessary, but not at the expense of research and innovation. Andrew Ng and Yann LeCun argued that a pause on developing or deploying generative AI technologies was unrealistic and counterproductive. They also called for more collaboration and transparency among researchers, governments and corporations to ensure the ethical and responsible use of generative AI.

Other critics of the open letter such as Arvind Narayanan, professor of computer science at Princeton, said on Twitter[55] that the letter *"further fuels AI hype and makes it harder to tackle real, already occurring AI harms"*, adding that he suspected that it will *"benefit the companies that it is supposed to regulate, and not society"*. Joanna Bryson, a professor of AI ethics at Hertie School in Berlin, also tweeted[56] that *"we don't need AI to be arbitrarily slowed, we need AI products to be safe. That involves following and documenting good practice, which requires regulation and audits"*. Emily Bender, professor of linguistics at the University of Washington, also tweeted[57] that *"the risks and harms have never been about 'too powerful AI'. Instead: They're about concentration of power in the hands of people, about reproducing systems of oppression, about damage to the information ecosystem, and about damage to the natural ecosystem (through profligate use of energy resources)"*. Indeed, what is most critical is not the technology as such, but rather who has control over the technology, how they use the technology and toward what objectives.

One of the first and most comprehensive, large-scale regulations came on April 2021 by the European Commission and the EU AI Act.[58] This is a draft proposal, and it is meant to be amended by members of the European Parliament and the governments of each EU member state. The proposal builds on existing EU law and the fundamental rights of fostering economic growth while offering safety and legal certainty for both companies and individuals. The EU AI Act puts forward a risk-based approach to evaluating the use of AI across tasks and domains. This risk-based approach ranges from identifying high-risk applications of AI that should be banned all the way to low-risk uses of AI where essentially no additional measures are required. The EU AI Act proposes ways to mitigate risk and harm proportionately to the risk identified for each AI technology, including conformity assessments before the AI technology goes to market or before it is deployed, so-called market monitoring mechanisms to see how an AI technology actually works in practice once it is rolled out for use, and outright bans of the technology. For example, social scoring systems that could lead to discrimination and unfair treatment or real-time remote biometric identification in publicly accessible spaces that could lead to privacy violations are examples of technology considered to be high-risk that could be banned.

The EU AI Act definitely sets a positive precedent for protecting both companies and individuals from possible harm that could be imparted by new generative AI technologies. However, just like other EU regulation such as the Digital Markets Act and the Digital Services Act[59] that are business model agnostic,[60] the EU AI Act targets all AI systems and classifies them according to their risk, as opposed to focusing on specific use cases and outcomes. This is problematic because not all AI technologies are generative and therefore their outcomes will differ vis-à-vis the digital services they may impact. Thus, instead of specifically defining generative AI technologies as being able to work on multiple tasks (e.g., classify words, images and video), across domains of use cases (e.g., administrative vs clinical) and produce versatile outputs, definitions remain generic and all-inclusive, meaning that even more narrow AI systems are subject to scrutiny.[61]

In addition, the EU AI Act designates as an AI "provider", *"a natural or legal person, public authority, agency or other body that develops an AI system or that has an AI system developed with a view to placing it on the market or putting it into service under its own name or trademark, whether for payment or free of charge"*.[62] That means that any developer of any AI system, large or small, including an individual, open-source developer that has just released a new machine learning technology on GitHub is subject to the Act and will have to comply with the same stringent obligations. Given the difficulty to comply with them, it can be expected that only large, resourceful actors (such as Google, Meta, Open AI) may field the costs to release a compliant AI technology. For open-source developers and many small, new startups, compliance will be prohibitively costly. Hence, regulatory acts such as the EU's AI Act will have the unintended consequence of spurring further concentration of power in the generative AI market. This is in direct opposition to the key objective of such regulatory acts that explicitly aim for an appropriate involvement of small- and medium-size enterprises to promote innovation and competitiveness in AI markets. Similar effects have already been established concerning the GDPR, with big tech companies reaping the benefits, while smaller organizations are negatively impacted.[63] In this sense, such regulatory acts threaten to undermine the efforts to infuse fair competition into the core of the digital economy.

Indeed, some have noted that two sections in the EU AI Act are particularly problematic for less resourceful actors, namely, data governance requirements and regulatory sandboxes.[64] In particular, the EU AI Act requires that AI technologies only use "high-quality", "free of bias" datasets that, as discussed in previous chapters, are impossible to achieve simply because all datasets reflect errors and biases of the historical practices of all organizations. No organization is immune to such errors and biases. Large, data-resourceful organizations may be in a better position to statistically minimize such errors, while smaller organizations are dependent on others to do so. Instead, some have noted that "documenting due diligence, best practice, and requirements for proportionate effort" is a more appropriate approach[65]. Similarly, regulatory sandboxes – *"established by one or more Member States competent authorities or the European Data Protection Supervisor [to] provide a controlled environment that facilitates the development, testing and validation of innovative AI systems for a limited time before their placement on the market or putting into service pursuant to a specific plan"*[66] – would still favor those with access to the right technological tools (including regulation compliant ones) to leverage the full potential of such sandboxes. These regulatory sandboxes would also likely be different across EU member states creating unequal competition.[67]

What is worrisome is that, exactly because of all the complex challenges faced by healthcare service providers all around the world, as discussed in Chapter 2, there is a steep increase in the demand for change and digital transformation. So much so, that smaller, less resourceful organizations become dependent on big tech. Indeed, a European Commission enterprise survey on the use of AI technologies shows that 60% of organizations report "purchased software or systems ready for use" as their AI strategy.[68] Thus, although generative AI technologies have the potential to reduce the costs of healthcare services by optimizing operations, improving the accuracy of diagnoses, reducing medical errors and streamlining administrative processes, there is a high cost of dependence on ready-made technologies usually provided by big tech companies.

This discussion is not meant to demonize large, resourceful organizations, most notably big tech companies, but rather to acknowledge the possibilities of winner-take-all dynamics exactly because of the scale of the digital platform ecosystems of these companies. As others have noted, big tech companies like Google, Meta, Microsoft, Apple, Amazon, Tencent and Baidu *"can bundle a broad range of digital services into a seamless data-driven offer that enables them to expand their reach into adjacent markets. The combination of economies of scale and scope, network effects, zero pricing, consumer behavioural biases, create new market dynamics with sudden radical decreases in competition ('tipping') and concentration of economic power around a few 'winner-*

takes-it-all/most' online platforms. Smaller businesses are increasingly dependent on a few very large online platforms to access digital markets and consumers. Innovative digital firms and start-ups find it difficult to compete with these very large online platforms. Their impact is compounded by the opacity and complexity of their large ecosystems, and the significant information advantage they have over business users".[69]

Given the possibilities of achieving winner-take-all markets, big tech companies have been criticized for lobbying against incorporating generative AI technologies in regulatory acts.[70] At times, such lobbying has been revealed in public as in the case of Google's Vice President Marian Croak, appointed to oversee Google's "Responsible AI". She argued that responsibility for compliance to regulation should not fall on big tech, but rather on "deployers", those organizations that modify AI technologies for specific tasks.[71] Others, including Microsoft, have signed an open letter sent to the Czech Presidency of the European Council that also places responsibility on "deployers" of AI systems as opposed to "developers" of such systems. "Such deployers can then require that developers and others within their supply chain make contractual commitments to assist them with compliance", the letter says.[72]

Certainly, deciding which responsibilities each actor in AI digital platform ecosystems should bear is key, and these signatories are correct in raising the issue of allocating responsibilities through contractual obligations. However, while deployers – for example, healthcare organizations that deploy a generative AI technology in their organization (these could be a consortium of hospitals or even a National Health Service) – should bear direct responsibility, the developers of these technologies should not be excluded from such responsibility. After all, they have the technological and human capabilities to better understand how these generative AI technologies work, better than any healthcare organization. Indeed, how many healthcare organizations, from hospitals to diagnostic centers, primary care, home care and specialist care organizations – but also pharmaceutical, insurance and other organizations in national and regional healthcare systems – are in a position to deploy such technologies on their own? Not even small tech startups can do so on their own, as they often depend on support, both financial and technological, by big tech companies.[73] Excluding big tech companies that develop generative AI technologies from responsibility creates a big hole in future regulation.

Evidently, the introduction of new generative AI technologies in healthcare is putting pressure on regulation. While there is a desire to bring new and innovative products to market quickly, there is also a need to ensure that these products are safe and effective for patients. The consequences of inadequate regulation can be significant, including harm to patients, loss of public trust, and even legal liability for companies and regulators. This is true both for countries or jurisdictions with less developed regulatory systems that may not have the resources, expertise or regulatory frameworks in place to adequately evaluate new technologies and ensure their safety and efficacy, but also for countries with strong regulatory systems. In both cases, because of the rapid pace of technological development, regulation may be outdated and unable to capture the negative effects of emergent technology even when first implemented.

The next subsection discusses some preliminary policy proposals put forward by academics and legal experts on how to regulate generative AI technology while ensuring innovation and fair competition among both small and large organizations. The proposals also consider the impact on user welfare, including both patients and individual healthcare service providers.

7.4 Technology Policy Proposals for Regulating Generative AI in Healthcare

7.4.1 *Increase Transparency Requirements for Ecosystem Actors*

Regulations like the EU AI Act definitely contain a wide range of disclosure obligations that offer a great start to regulating generative AI in healthcare. However, transparency requirements for all ecosystem actors, including ecosystem orchestrators that may provide the core technology, ecosystem complementors that provide complementary technologies and professional users such as hospitals that may deploy these technologies.

Specifically, ecosystem orchestrators and complementors, as providers of the core and complementary technologies, should be required to report on the infrastructure characteristics of their technology, including system architecture, use of computing resources, datasheets for datasets, development methods and use of third-party technologies, validation and testing and a number of performance metrics. Such performance metrics may include the level of accuracy, robustness and resilience against cybersecurity threats, human oversight and potential biases, among others,[74] but also the technology's greenhouse gas (GHG) emissions, especially as organizations aim toward a net zero commitment.[75] In addition, ecosystem orchestrators and complementors should be required to report on any incidents and mitigation strategies concerning harmful content or foreseeable sources of risk to health and safety, fundamental rights and discrimination. These risks need to be continuously evaluated, especially as technologies are updated, integrated with new complementary technologies or deployed in new organizational settings with new datasets.

Professional users like hospitals or other healthcare organizations should be required to disclose where they deployed which technology, to perform which task and while using which datasets. They should also report on which parts of outcomes are generated by these technologies or adapted based on their output, as opposed to outcomes produced by human experts or other more conventional technologies. This is important to adequately inform users, including patients, of whether outcomes were synthetically generated or not. While the added value of such information may be limited in some tasks and domains (e.g., cases where no patient data is involved and where there are no direct impacts on patient outcomes), such information is arguably crucial in any cases involving patient data and informed consent over their use. Professional users may use such a disclosure as a warning signal and engage in additional monitoring and risk management. Failure to adhere to such transparency obligations should be subject to fines and other conformance violations penalties (e.g., restricted access to technologies and data).

Even non-professional users like patients or communities should be required to disclose how they intend to use these technologies. There have already been many reported cases of so called "deepfakes", that is, media, including text, audio, photos and video that have been digitally manipulated to replace real people and their actions, but also events with fake ones.[76] In healthcare this could be particularly problematic, as non-professional users may present false evidence to get access to data and content that they would not have otherwise been able to access. Exactly because they do not have to conform to the same standards and regulatory obligations as professional users they may engage in unscrupulous behavior and spread misinformation to manipulate decision-making. There is plenty of evidence of such behaviors emerging from the COVID-19 pandemic and the misinformation spread around the use of vaccines.[77] Safety measures should be built in publicly available generative AI technologies to identify cases of misinformation by non-professional users, including potentially malicious posts and deepfakes, with traditional civil and criminal charges brought forward. Failing to conform should be subject to significant financially fines, something which will provide greater incentives to refrain from harmful content propagation. Research into safe and responsible AI is already advancing technical mechanisms of detecting such harmful content and unsafe use.[78]

The potential misuse of generative AI technologies for disinformation, manipulation and harm is probably the biggest challenge faced by regulatory bodies. This is particularly true for generative AI technologies offered as standalone software or integrated into widely used digital platforms like Microsoft's Office 365. Monitoring and auditing such potential misuse would require coordination between all ecosystem actors including non-professional users in a polycentric governance structure. Such a structure would combine a generic, crowd-based monitoring center and a specialized, ecosystem-specific monitoring center. The generic, crowd-based monitoring center would use non-professional users to flag problematic content and give notice. These users could be organized into trusted groups, including individual patients, independent technology communities and other social groups (e.g., ethics group) that can function as a crowd-based content monitoring team. They could experiment with different prompts with the technology and see if they manage to generate harmful or otherwise problematic content. They could also scan the Internet for tools to circumvent content moderation policies. These trusted groups would send a notice to other ecosystem actors, including the orchestrator, complementors and professional users. The specialized, ecosystem-specific monitoring center would then respond to the notices submitted by the trusted groups. Their responses would be to modify the technology, to block specific outputs and any tools that can circumvent content moderation policies. Such a polycentric governance structure would help complement current monitoring systems.

7.4.2   *Risk Management Throughout the Development Process*

As noted in the previous proposal, ecosystem orchestrators and complementors should be accountable for the initial design, development, use of data and other choices regarding the infrastructure and neural network of the generative AI technologies. However, risk management does not stop there. These technologies – like the digital platforms discussed in Chapter 4 – can have varied technology architectures, from fully open to fully closed. As such, researchers have proposed that generative AI technologies be released "gradiently" – from access to the model itself, access to components that enable further risk analysis and access to components that enable model replication.[79] The key objective would be to trade off the value of public scrutiny with the risk of misuse and harm in the case of fully open, public releases.[80] Ecosystem orchestrators and complementors should manage such risk by following a staged release of the aforementioned components, starting by providing access only to safe and responsible AI researchers and selected stakeholders. This adds a community-based risk management strategy that would help to institute codes of conduct, as an extension to the regulation.[81] Most importantly, these community-based risk management strategy will help to audit the concentration of power to large, resourceful organizations in successive stages of release, including updates to the core model itself.

As part of the audits on the development process, ecosystem orchestrators and complementors should show evidence of data curation policies, for example, representativeness and approximate balance between protected groups. In particular, ecosystem orchestrators and complementors should pro-actively audit the training dataset for misrepresentations of protected groups, in ways proportionate to their size and the type of training material (internally curated data vs. data scraped from the Internet) and implement feasible mitigation measures. Some have also suggested that real-world training data should be complemented with synthetic data to balance historical and societal biases contained in online sources. "For example, content concerning professions historically reserved for one gender (nurse; doctor) could be automatically copied and any female first names or images exchanged by male ones, and vice versa, creating a training corpus with more gender-neutral professions for text and image generation".[82]

7.4.3 *Implement Regulatory Mechanisms that are Adaptive and Scalable*

Generative AI technologies are *"unsafe by default"*,[83] meaning that, by design, they give rise to a number of risks, as already discussed. Many of these risks are not generated by malicious actors, but rather by the possibilities imparted by the technology itself. Our biggest problem is control: humans want to retain absolute power and control over AI technologies that are more powerful than us.[84] So, regulation, including the proposals made in the previous sections, aims at incentivizing actors to control the AI technology to perform in the best interests of those actors. But as previous experience with similar disruptive technology has shown, if the performance of that technology is measured on the basis of a crude proxy (e.g., an incentive to maximize X interest), the technology may cause tremendous harm solely in trying to achieve that proxy. For example, generative AI technology developed to accelerate drug discovery could end up designing chemical weapons.

These risks are aggravated by the fact that much generative AI technology is general-purpose with the ability to integrate with other AI systems. Thus, risks become increasingly systemic and complex. It is exactly the acknowledgment of such systemic risk that informed the risk-based approach of the EU AI Act and more recently the Canadian AI and Data Act.[85] Others seem to follow suit.[86] While placing emphasis on risk is important, the focus seems to be primarily on product safety. As others have noted, rather than address the broader, more systemic and longer-term implications of unsafe AI technologies, current regulation primarily targets the immediate risks to individual users. "Considering the noteworthy risks AI poses to social and political institutions, this individual-centric regulatory approach is inappropriate".[87]

This final proposal calls for the implementation of regulatory mechanisms that continue to adapt and scale to mitigate large-scale, systemic risk. The previous two proposals focus primarily on preventative and interventionist mechanisms, while this proposal calls for treatment after the fact. Since it is impossible to know in advance emergent risks, regulation should – by design – allow for the option to make reversible decisions. Such flexibility would help to accommodate new data and learning about the evolving nature of the technology and its applications. Likewise, regulation should incorporate mechanisms that can scale as AI technologies scale to perform more complex tasks and diverse domains. Regulatory adaptability and scalability is common in the regulation of pharmaceuticals, aviation and cybersecurity[88] and should be no different with AI regulation. AI regulatory adaptability and scalability requires a shift away from relying on rigid written rules and cumbersome compliance mechanisms, and toward building new regulatory technology. In other words, AI regulation "will require almost as much or more AI than the AI targets of regulation themselves".[89]

In conclusion, the performance of generative AI technologies scales exponentially,[90] something that makes it very difficult to predict the emergent capabilities of these technologies and, consequentially, the risks lurking underneath every exponential jump. "Even if a technology is deployed by an actor with good intentions and substantial oversight, good outcomes are not guaranteed".[91] Regulators are up against what seems to be an impossible task: protecting against unknown risks, arising from unknown capabilities. The stakes are high, especially in healthcare, and all ecosystem actors need to coordinate their efforts to ensure such risks are better understood and mitigated.

Notes

1 https://blogs.microsoft.com/blog/2023/03/06/introducing-microsoft-dynamics-365-copilot/
2 https://workspace.google.com/blog/product-announcements/generative-ai
3 https://techcrunch.com/2022/12/31/how-china-is-building-a-parallel-generative-ai-universe
4 https://github.com/steven2358/awesome-generative-ai
5 Gary Marcus, Sam Altman and Christina Montgomery testimonies to the US Senate Subcommittee: https://time.com/6280372/sam-altman-chatgpt-regulate-ai/
6 See https://www.crn.com/news/cloud/aws-microsoft-alibaba-led-iaas-cloud-services-in-2020-gartner
7 Goodfellow, I.J., 2014. On Distinguishability Criteria for Estimating Generative Models. *arXiv preprint arXiv:1412.6515.*
8 Rosenfeld. R. 2000. Two Decades of Statistical Language Modelling: Where Do We Go From Here? *Proc. IEEE 88*, 8 (2000), pp. 1270–1278.
9 https://aiindex.stanford.edu/report/
10 See as recent blog by Bill Gates that refers to exactly this possibility https://www.gatesnotes.com/The-Age-of-AI-Has-Begun
11 https://blogs.microsoft.com/blog/2023/03/16/introducing-microsoft-365-copilot-your-copilot-for-work/
12 The World Health Organization estimates a projected shortfall of 10 million health workers by 2030 https://www.who.int/health-topics/health-workforce
13 Xu, I.R., Van Booven, D.J., Goberdhan, S., Breto, A., Porto, J., Alhusseini, M., Algohary, A., Stoyanova, R., Punnen, S., Mahne, A. and Arora, H., 2023. Generative Adversarial Networks Can Create High Quality Artificial Prostate Cancer Magnetic Resonance Images. *Journal of Personalized Medicine, 13*(3), p. 547.
14 Shanehsazzadeh, A., Bachas, S., McPartlon, M., Kasun, G., Sutton, J.M., Steiger, A.K., Shuai, R., Kohnert, C., Rakocevic, G., Gutierrez, J.M. and Chung, C., 2023. Unlocking De Novo Antibody Design with Generative Artificial Intelligence. *bioRxiv*, pp. 2023–01.
15 https://www.benevolent.com/
16 https://www.mendelian.co/
17 https://www.cogitotech.com/
18 See for example Babylon Health's AI Symptom Checker. https://www.babylonhealth.com/en-gb/ai/learn-more
19 See https://ai-derm.com/
20 https://www.medimaging.net/ultrasound/articles/294792215/ai-algorithm-reads-ultrasound-images-from-hand-held-devices-and-smartphone.html
21 Castelvecchi, D., 2016. Can We Open the Black Box of AI?. *Nature News, 538*(7623), p. 20.
22 Miotto, R., Li, L., Kidd, B.A. and Dudley, J.T., 2016. Deep Patient: An Unsupervised Representation to Predict the Future of Patients from the Electronic Health Records. *Scientific Reports, 6*(1), pp. 1–10.
23 https://www.technologyreview.com/2017/04/11/5113/the-dark-secret-at-the-heart-of-ai/
24 Caruana, R., Lou, Y., Gehrke, J., Koch, P., Sturm, M. and Elhadad, N., 2015, August. Intelligible Models for Healthcare: Predicting Pneumonia Risk and Hospital 30-day Readmission. In *Proceedings of the 21th ACM SIGKDD International Conference on Knowledge Discovery and Data Mining* (pp. 1721–1730).

25 DARPA. 2016. *Broad Agency Announcement: Explainable Artificial Intelligence (XAI)*. DARPA-BAA-16-53. August 10, 2016. Available at https://www.darpa.mil/program/explainable-artificial-intelligence

26 Bender, E.M., Gebru, T., McMillan-Major, A. and Shmitchell, S., 2021, March. On the Dangers of Stochastic Parrots: Can Language Models Be Too Big?. In *Proceedings of the 2021 ACM Conference on Fairness, Accountability, and Transparency* (pp. 610–623).

27 World Bank. 2018. Individuals Using the Internet. (2018). https://data.worldbank.org/indicator/IT.NET.USER.ZS?end=2017&locations=US&start=2015; Pew. 2018. Internet/Broadband Fact Sheet. (2 2018). https://www.pewinternet.org/fact-sheet/internet-broadband

28 Ibid. p. 614.

29 Obermeyer, Z., Powers, B., Vogeli, C. and Mullainathan, S., 2019. Dissecting Racial Bias in an Algorithm Used to Manage the Health of Populations. *Science*, 366(6464), pp. 447–453.

30 López-Cabrera, J.D., Orozco-Morales, R., Portal-Diaz, J.A., Lovelle-Enríquez, O. and Pérez-Díaz, M., 2021. Current Limitations to Identify COVID-19 using Artificial Intelligence with Chest X-ray Imaging. *Health and Technology*, 11(2), pp. 411–424.

31 https://www.healthcaredive.com/news/generative-AI-healthcare-gpt-potential/648104/

32 Fenech, M., Strukelj, N. and Buston, O., 2018. Ethical, Social, and Political Challenges of Artificial Intelligence in Health. *London: Wellcome Trust Future Advocacy*, 12.

33 Strubell, E. Ganesh, A., and McCallum, A. 2019. Energy and Policy Considerations for Deep Learning in NLP. In *Proceedings of the 57th Annual Meeting of the Association for Computational Linguistics*, 3645–3650.

34 Bender, E.M., Gebru, T., McMillan-Major, A. and Shmitchell, S., 2021, March. On the Dangers of Stochastic Parrots: Can Language Models Be Too Big?. In *Proceedings of the 2021 ACM Conference on Fairness, Accountability, and Transparency* (pp. 610–623).

35 Nori, H., King, N., McKinney, S.M., Carignan, D. and Horvitz, E., 2023. Capabilities of GPT-4 on Medical Challenge Problems. *arXiv preprint arXiv:2303.13375*.

36 OpenAI (2023). GPT-4 technical report. Technical report, OpenAI. https://cdn.openai.com/papers/gpt-4.pdf

37 Eloundou, T., Manning, S., Mishkin, P. and Rock, D., 2023. Gpts are Gpts: An Early Look at the Labor Market Impact Potential of Large Language Models. *arXiv preprint arXiv:2303.10130*.

38 Rai, A., Constantinides, P. and Sarker, S., 2019. Next Generation Digital Platforms:: Toward Human-AI Hybrids. *Mis Quarterly*, 43(1), pp. iii–ix.

39 Autor, D., Mindell, D. A., and Reynolds, E. B. (2022). *The Work of the Future: Building Better Jobs in an Age of Intelligent Machines*. The MIT Press.

40 Obviously the compute power required would have energy costs and environmental implications as discussed earlier. However, what is more costly, machines with humans or machines only?

41 Ahmed, N., Wahed, M., and Thompson, N.C. 2023. The growing Influence of Industry in AI Research: Industry is Gaining Control Over the Technology's Future. *Science*, Vol 379, Issue 6635, pp. 884–886.

42 https://www.deepmind.com/blog/deepminds-health-team-joins-google-health

43 https://www.deepmind.com/research/highlighted-research/alphafold

44 https://news.microsoft.com/2023/04/17/microsoft-and-epic-expand-strategic-collaboration-with-integration-of-azure-openai-service/

45 https://www.fiercehealthcare.com/health-tech/how-amazons-one-medical-deal-could-boost-its-healthcare-ambitions-and-heat-competition

46 See, for example, how DeepMind handled data from the Royal Free Foundation NHS Trust https://www.theguardian.com/technology/2017/jul/03/google-deepmind-16m-patient-royal-free-deal-data-protection-act; See also more recent cases of the use of UK NHS data by Amazon, and US health data by Facebook and Apple https://www.wired.co.uk/article/google-apple-amazon-nhs-health-data

47 The leaked memo was posted on May 4, 2023 on SemiAnalysis https://www.semianalysis.com/p/google-we-have-no-moat-and-neither?utm_source=www.theneurondaily.com&utm_medium=referral&utm_campaign=google-memo-leaked

48 Hardin, G., 1968. The Tragedy of the Commons: The Population Problem Has No Technical Solution; It Requires a Fundamental Extension in Morality. *Science*, 162(3859), pp.1243–1248. See how the tragedy of the commons apply to technologies in healthcare in Constantinides, P.,

2012. *Perspectives and implications for the development of information infrastructures.* IGI Global; Constantinides, P. and Barrett, M., 2015. Information Infrastructure Development and Governance as Collective Action. *Information Systems Research*, 26(1), pp. 40–56. Also see how it applies to platform ecosystems in Cennamo, C. and Santaló, J., 2019. Generativity Tension and Value Creation in Platform Ecosystems. *Organization Science*, 30(3), pp. 617–641; O'Mahony, S. and Karp, R., 2020. From Proprietary to Collective Governance: How Do Platform Participation Strategies Evolve?. *Strategic Management Journal.*

49 Ljungberg, J., 2000. Open Source Movements as a Model for Organising. *European Journal of Information Systems*, 9(4), pp. 208–216.

50 See list of benevolent dictators here https://en.wikipedia.org/wiki/Benevolent_dictator_for_life

51 See open letter and signatories here https://futureoflife.org/open-letter/pause-giant-ai-experiments/

52 https://futureoflife.org/

53 For example, see fake images of Obama and Merkel enjoying a summer holiday https://www.ndtv.com/offbeat/ai-generated-images-of-barack-obama-and-angela-merkel-enjoying-vacation-on-a-beach-amazes-internet-3878630; but also fake images of Donald Trump fighting police https://www.pbs.org/newshour/politics/fake-ai-images-of-putin-trump-being-arrested-spread-online

54 See full discussion here https://www.youtube.com/watch?v=BY9KV8uCtj4

55 https://twitter.com/random_walker/status/1641077455178833920

56 https://twitter.com/j2bryson/status/1640997159964139520

57 https://twitter.com/emilymbender/status/1640922978165882880

58 Proposal for a Regulation of the European Parliament and of the Council Laying Down Harmonised Rules on Artificial Intelligence (Artificial Intelligence Act) and Amending Certain Union Legislative Acts. Available at https://eur-lex.europa.eu/legal-content/EN/TXT/?qid=1623335154975&uri=CELEX%3A52021PC0206

59 See extensive discussion in Cabral, L., Haucap, J., Parker, G., Petropoulos, G., Valletti, T.M. and Van Alstyne, M.W., 2021. The EU Digital Markets Act: A Report From a Panel of Economic Experts. Cabral, L., Haucap, J., Parker, G., Petropoulos, G., Valletti, T. & Van Alstyne, M., The EU Digital Markets Act, Publications Office of the European Union, Luxembourg.

60 See criticism on the DMA's business model agnosticism in Cennamo, C., Kretschmer, T., Constantinides, P., Alaimo, C. and Santaló, J., 2023. Digital Platforms Regulation: An Innovation-Centric View of the EU's Digital Markets Act. *Journal of European Competition Law & Practice*, 14(1), pp. 44–51; Constantinides, P., 2022. Regulating Digital Platforms: Business Models, Technology Architectures, and Governance Rules (2022). *Competition Policy International: TechReg Chronicle*, 23, pp. 30–35, January 2022.

61 Hacker, P., Engel, A. and Mauer, M., 2023. Regulating Chatgpt and Other Large Generative AI Models. *arXiv preprint arXiv:2302.02337.*

62 Article 3 of the EU AI Act, Available at https://eur-lex.europa.eu/legal-content/EN/TXT/?qid=1623335154975&uri=CELEX%3A52021PC0206

63 Geradin, D., Karanikioti, T. and Katsifis, D., 2021. GDPR Myopia: How a Well-intended Regulation Ended Up Favouring Large Online Platforms-the Case Of Ad Tech. *European Competition Journal*, 17(1), pp. 47–92; Peukert, C., Bechtold, S., Batikas, M. and Kretschmer, T., 2022. Regulatory Spillovers and Data Governance: Evidence from the GDPR. *Marketing Science*, 41(4), pp. 746–768.

64 Haataja, M. and Bryson, J.J., 2022. Reflections on the EU's AI Act and How we Could Make It Even Better. *Competition Policy International: TechReg Chronicle*, 24.

65 Ibid.

66 Article 53(1) of the EU AI Act, Available at https://eur-lex.europa.eu/legal-content/EN/TXT/?qid=1623335154975&uri=CELEX%3A52021PC0206

67 Yordanova, K., 2022. The EU AI Act-Balancing Human Rights and Innovation Through Regulatory Sandboxes and Standardization. *Competition Policy International: TechReg Chronicle*, 24.

68 European Commission, Directorate-General for Communications Networks, Content and Technology, *European Enterprise Survey on the Use of Technologies Based on Artificial Intelligence: Final Report*, Publications Office, 2020, https://data.europa.eu/doi/10.2759/759368

69 Cabral, L., Haucap, J., Parker, G., Petropoulos, G., Valletti, T.M. and Van Alstyne, M.W., 2021. The EU Digital Markets Act: A Report From a Panel of Economic Experts. Cabral, L., Haucap, J., Parker, G., Petropoulos, G., Valletti, T. and Van Alstyne, M., The EU Digital Markets Act, Publications Office of the European Union, Luxembourg, page 6.

70 See report by the Corporate Europe Observatory, 2023. "The Lobbying Ghost in the Machine: Big Tech's covert defanging of Europe's AI Act", February 2023. https://corporateeurope.org/sites/default/files/2023-02/The%20Lobbying%20Ghost%20in%20the%20Machine.pdf

71 See the position statement by Marian Croak, vice president, engineering, responsible AI and human centered technology at Google here https://www.youtube.com/watch?v=uvaUQg_q2Ho

72 See open letter here: https://www.spcr.cz/images/Open_letter_on_the_proposed_regulation_of_artificial_intelligence_FIN20221107_125114.pdf

73 See report by the Corporate Europe Observatory, 2023. "The Lobbying Ghost in the Machine: Big Tech's covert defanging of Europe's AI Act", February 2023. https://corporateeurope.org/sites/default/files/2023-02/The%20Lobbying%20Ghost%20in%20the%20Machine.pdf

74 See Haataja, M. and Bryson, J.J., 2022. Reflections on the EU's AI Act and How we Could Make It Even Better. *Competition Policy International: TechReg Chronicle, 24.*

75 https://www.un.org/en/climatechange/net-zero-coalition

76 https://www.techtarget.com/whatis/definition/deepfake

77 Loomba, S., de Figueiredo, A., Piatek, S.J., de Graaf, K. and Larson, H.J., 2021. Measuring the Impact of COVID-19 Vaccine Misinformation on Vaccination Intent in the UK and USA. *Nature* Human Behaviour, *5*(3), pp. 337–348.

78 Brown, T., Mann, B., Ryder, N., Subbiah, M., Kaplan, J.D., Dhariwal, P., Neelakantan, A., Shyam, P., Sastry, G., Askell, A. and Agarwal, S., 2020. Language Models are Few-Shot Learners. *Advances in Neural Information Processing Systems, 33,* pp. 1877–1901; Gongane, V.U., Munot, M.V. and Anuse, A.D., 2022. Detection and Moderation of Detrimental Content on Social Media Platforms: Current Status and Future Directions. *Social Network Analysis and Mining, 12*(1), p. 129; Rando, J., Paleka, D., Lindner, D., Heim, L. and Tramèr, F., 2022. Red-Teaming the Stable Diffusion Safety Filter. *arXiv preprint arXiv:2210.04610.*

79 Solaiman, I., 2023. The Gradient of Generative AI Release: Methods and Considerations. *arXiv preprint arXiv:2302.04844;*

80 Solaiman, I., 2023. The Gradient of Generative AI Release: Methods and Considerations. *arXiv preprint arXiv:2302.04844;* Solaiman, I., Brundage, M., Clark, J., Askell, A., Herbert-Voss, A., Wu, J., Radford, A., Krueger, G., Kim, J.W., Kreps, S. and McCain, M., 2019. Release Strategies and the Social Impacts of Language Models. *arXiv preprint arXiv:1908.09203.*

81 Hacker, P., Engel, A. and Mauer, M., 2023. Regulating Chatgpt and Other Large Generative AI Models. *arXiv preprint arXiv:2302.02337.*

82 Ibid.

83 Kolt, N., 2023. Algorithmic Black Swans. *Washington University Law Review, 101.*

84 Russell, S., 2019. *Human Compatible: Artificial Intelligence and the Problem of Control.* Penguin.

85 https://ised-isde.canada.ca/site/innovation-better-canada/en/artificial-intelligence-and-data-act-aida-companion-document

86 See for example a discussion of China's AI policies https://carnegieendowment.org/2022/01/04/china-s-new-ai-governance-initiatives-shouldn-t-be-ignored-pub-86127

87 Kolt, N., 2023. Algorithmic Black Swans. *Washington University Law Review, 101.*

88 Ibid.

89 Hadfield, G.K., 2017. *Rules for a Flat World: Why Humans Invented Law and How to Reinvent it for a Complex Global Economy.* Oxford University Press.

90 Kaplan, J., McCandlish, S., Henighan, T., Brown, T.B., Chess, B., Child, R., Gray, S., Radford, A., Wu, J. and Amodei, D., 2020. Scaling Laws for Neural Language Models. *arXiv preprint arXiv:2001.08361.*

91 Bowman, S., 2022, May. The Dangers of Underclaiming: Reasons for Caution When Reporting How NLP Systems Fail. In *Proceedings of the 60th Annual Meeting of the Association for Computational Linguistics (Volume 1: Long Papers)* (pp. 7484–7499).

Index

Note: **Bold** page numbers refer to tables and *italic* page numbers refer to figures.